Start Line
Running for a better life

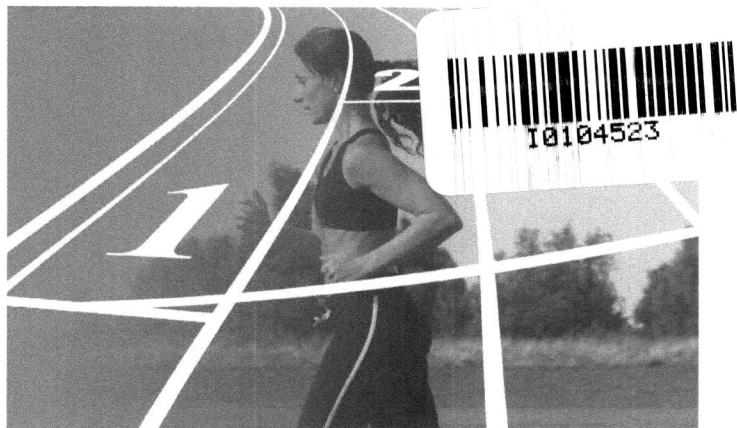

I0104523

Martin Haigh &
Geoff Cumber

Foreword by Steve Cram CBE

Fisher King Publishing

Fitness matters and helps with...

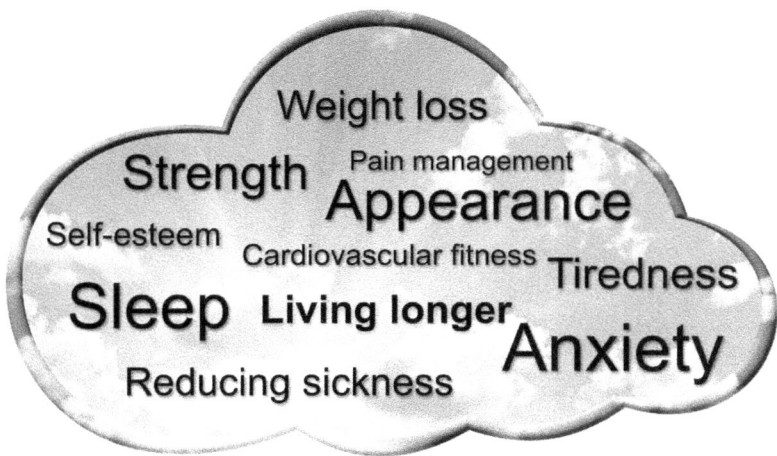

Weight loss

Strength
Pain management
Appearance

Self-esteem
Cardiovascular fitness
Tiredness

Sleep
Living longer
Anxiety

Reducing sickness

Start Line
Copyright © Martin Haigh & Geoff Cumber 2015
ISBN 978-1-910406-12-0

Published by
Fisher King Publishing
The Studio
Arthington Lane
Pool-in-Wharfedale
LS21 1JZ
England

Contents

Contents

Foreword

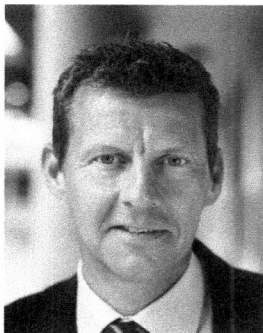

Running has been a
major part of my life since
childhood. Having spent
many years working hard to win some major
titles on the track, I have always recognised
the importance of regular exercise. I am
delighted to recommend this book by Martin
and Geoff, which offers a wealth of useful
advice to runners.

Steve Cram CBE

Abstract

Many people believe they are generally healthy but, actually, they have an opportunity to improve their fitness even more. Our physical well-being can be improved and this, in turn, can improve our emotional wellbeing.

However, according to recent statistics from the NHS Information Centre for Health and Social Care*, more than 30 per cent of men and women said they were sedentary for six or more hours daily. The report also showed that many individuals are trying to increase their physical activity levels. Despite these positive steps in the right direction, more needs to be done to encourage active lifestyles. Sport England, for example, launched 'This Girl Can' campaign in January 2015, in an attempt to encourage more women into sport. This comes out of research revealing that there are significantly fewer women than men who engage in sport on a regular basis.

There is mounting evidence to support the notion that regular exercise is an essential component of a healthy lifestyle, and that those who do lead active lifestyles have a reduced risk of developing a range of health concerns. It is clear that people (especially the young) are spending many hours per day using their mobile devices. This indicates a tendency for people to bend forward and look down for long periods and this action, known as 'Text Neck', can put additional strain on a whole range of muscles, causing stiffness.

Research from The University of Cambridge**, released in January 2015, shows that a 'lack of exercise' could be killing twice as many people as 'obesity'. This 12-year study of more than 300,000 people, in Europe, suggests that about 676,000 deaths each year were down to inactivity. This is compared with 337,000 deaths from carrying too much weight. They concluded that exercise was beneficial for people of any weight. People who exercise are less likely to get ill and generally live longer. However, finding the motivation to get active can be quite challenging for some. Physical activity does not have to be vigorous and everyone and anyone, from young children and teenagers through to pregnant women and the elderly, can incorporate at least some form of exercise, even brisk walking, into their daily routine.

Regular exercise in old age has as powerful an effect on life expectancy as giving up smoking and elderly people who exercise 'live five years longer' than those with more sedentary lifestyles. This comes out of a report *** published in the British Journal of Sports Medicine, in May 2015, following the analysis of 5,700 men, with an average age of 73, in Norway.

Whilst this book uncovers the physiological advantages of running, it's not just about the physical benefits. Being involved in running (even at a relatively sedentary level) gives us a feeling of well-being to the point where we are much better equipped to handle challenges in life. Running gives us renewed vigour and helps us to enjoy life into old age. Grandparents want to be able to enjoy picking up their grandchildren without being out of breath.

It is written to help you discover the fundamentals of running and fitness and there are many references and signposts to associated helpful websites and articles. Start Line is written in a modular fashion and, whilst, there is a continuous flavour running through the book, the chapters are 'stand alone'. Therefore, the reader can dip in and out as required. This book goes beyond running as a fitness mechanism and covers the broader topics of flexibility, strength training, high intensity training (HIT), swimming and cycling.

There are specific chapters on topics such as pain management, women's running and access for the disabled and the content of these chapters has been ratified by experts in the particular field.

Start Line is written in an easy to read style which will encourage readers to continue browsing and learning more about running fitness. Throughout the book, you will see *valuable* 'Authors' Tips' from Martin and Geoff's vast experience.

Enjoy the read and we hope this motivates you to get out there and discover the benefits that improved fitness brings.

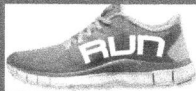

Wherever you see this image: ...there will be a top tip from the author's.

* NHS Information Centre for Health and Social Care 2008.

** Prof Ulf Ekelund, University of Cambridge, 2015

*** Increases in physical activity is as important as smoking cessation for reduction in total mortality in elderly men: 12 years of follow-up of the Oslo II study, by I Holme and SA Anderssen. Published in the British Journal of Sports Medicine 2015; 49:743-748 doi:10.1136/bjsports-2014-094522.

Acknowledgements

We are delighted that you have chosen to read this book and we hope that it gives you much pleasure. This publication has been greatly enhanced with the help of fellow runners, especially members of Halifax Harriers AC and the athletic associations who have provided invaluable guidance ard advice.

We would also like to acknowledge the health professionals who have provided comprehensive, factual advice. We wish to acknowledge the support of Bruce Fitzgerald Photography for many of the images in this book and the organisations that have kindly granted permission to reproduce images and content. We are grateful to Louise Clarke, of Louise Clarke Communications, for making editorial suggestions in the early days of the project and for proofreading the final manuscript. We also highly appreciate the advice given on chapter '0, by Jo Hague, Deputy Headteacher at Ravenscliffe High School and Sports College, Halifax. Without the expert guidance of our publisher, Fisher King Publishing and the motivatior of their CEO, Rick Armstrong, this publication would not have been possible.

Finally, we are indebted to our wives, Melanie and Sarah for their patience, love and encouragement during the writing and publication of this book.

Martin Haigh & Geoff Cumber

Lets Get Physical

So what are the physical benefits of running?

Our circumstances often change

During our lifetime, our circumstances can change. We may be looking for employment or elected to take early retirement. Our friends sometimes move away from the area, our children become less dependent on us and eventually flee the nest. We might separate from a partner, get divorced or our partners might pass away. When life circumstances, of this magnitude, change we look for substitutes. Fitness is a highly productive, valuable way to help us balance change or transition in our lives.

The human body is going through a process of change

Throughout life, changes occur in our skin, skeletal system, muscular system and immune system. Changes also occur in our neurology, digestive system and cardiovascular organs. The above two key change systems build up pressure and can show up as anxiety, depression, alcoholism and other substance abuse. Poor posture, fatigue, lack of sleep, excessive muscle wastage, obesity, poor eating habits, lack of control, low self-esteem and lack of confidence can also be exhibited.

Exercise can bring many physical and emotional benefits and you do not have to be Usain Bolt to realise them. Sully Sullenberger (the pilot who safely landed a plane on the

Hudson River) said: "I am not a 'good' runner but I am better than someone who does not do it at all!" The authors: Martin Haigh and Geoff Cumber have found that running, and other fitness activities, have changed their lives for the better. People cannot believe how young they look for their age and they have the energy to relate to young people. Of course, there are other benefits of running which are not related to your health, such as being socially inclusive. Just putting on your shoes and going for a run or a brisk walk is the most convenient and inexpensive form of exercise we know.

So how do we respond to the above changes?
Dealing with circumstantial issues – running and exercise are the body's inherent mechanism for self-gratification and can significantly improve a person's self-worth. Running makes us feel better, look better, relax more and behave in a positive way towards the outside world. Running is a great way to meet new friends and start long-lasting friendships with positive people. It is a way to help us appreciate the countryside and the many beautiful places that exist around us. Ever had that niggling problem that you just couldn't find the answer to; well, running allows our sub-conscious mind to be working on our problems whilst we are out enjoying the scenery and camaraderie. You may often find that when you get back from your run, your friendly sub-conscious has solved that niggling problem for you and you feel better as a result.

Improving our emotional and physical health – running can help us to strengthen our bones (especially women), improve our cardiovascular system, improve concentration and mental *enerally speaking, exercise brings with it very positive benefits. However, before you start running it is advisable to visit your GP in order to have a basic medical check. Your GP will, most likely, test for heart conditions, cardiovascular efficiency, blood pressure, etc.*

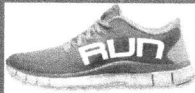

toughness and control weight which may lead to increased longevity and a slowing down of the ageing process.

It probably comes as no surprise that exercise can bring many physical benefits. These benefits will be very different for each individual but typically, exercise can:

Reduce the Risk of Heart Disease
It is quite normal to be slightly breathless after walking up three flights of stairs but it is not good to be struggling for breath at the top of the stairs or needing to stop to complete the climb. A lack of fitness can lead to high blood pressure and increasing breathlessness. Running physically strengthens your heart and increases lung capacity which, in turn, improves the flow of oxygen and blood throughout your body, helping to reduce the risk of heart disease. This is because your heart is a muscle and all muscles need to be exercised and supplied with blood in order to function properly.

Reduce your Cholesterol level
Cholesterol is a waxy, fat-like substance made in the liver

and other cells. It is also found in certain foods, such as dairy products, eggs, and meat. We all need a certain amount of cholesterol, but too much can lead to hardening of the arteries, heart disease and related complications. There are two main forms of cholesterol, LDL (Low Density Lipoprotein) and HDL (High Density Lipoprotein). LDL cholesterol is often referred to as bad cholesterol because too much is unhealthy. HDL is often referred to as 'good cholesterol'. It has been shown that running (together with sensible eating) can control the levels of cholesterol in your body. Please see Case Study 1.

Lower Blood Pressure

Research (Bloodpressureuk.org) has proven that running lowers blood pressure. According to the experts, lower blood pressure often occurs in runners because the arteries become more relaxed and flexible. Controlled blood pressure means that you reduce the risk of certain health conditions; such as: heart disease, stroke, kidney damage and complications with the eyes. If you have high blood pressure, your doctor or nurse may suggest that you try to become more active to lower it. However, you may be worried that regular exercise will increase your blood pressure to dangerous levels.

Physical activity can cause your blood pressure to rise for a short time. However, when you stop the activity, your blood pressure should soon return to normal. The quicker it does this, the fitter you are likely to be. Most people with high blood pressure should be able to increase their physical activity levels quite safely. However, if your blood pressure is relatively high, your health professional may prefer to help you lower it with medication before you start an exercise programme. If your blood pressure is very high, you should not start any new activity without first consulting your health professional.

Table 1 gives a general idea of what levels you need to be concerned about, but bear in mind that every person is different, and your health professional may advise you accordingly.

Blood Pressure level	General ability to be more active
Below 90/60	You may have low blood pressure. Speak to your health professional before starting any new exercise
90/60 – 140/90	It is probably safe to be more active, and it will help to keep your blood pressure in this ideal blood pressure range
140/90 – 179/99	It should be safe to start increasing your physical activity to help lower your high blood pressure
180/100 – 199/109	Speak to your health professional before starting any new exercise
200/100 or above	Do not start any new activity – speak to your health professional

Table 1 Blood Pressure levels

What do the numbers mean? Each blood pressure level has a pair of numbers. The first number (systolic or highest blood pressure), shows the pressure when the heart is squeezing and pushing the blood round the body. The second number (diastolic or lowest blood pressure) is the pressure between heart beats and gives the best idea of your risk of having a stroke or heart attack.

To be safe, it is always a good idea to get professional advice before you start any new physical activity.

Support Weight control

A popular side-effect of running is weight loss, or weight control. Keep a journal of what you eat and follow a good runners' diet and you are likely to lose weight. You will also be able to use running to keep the weight off. Weight control, a healthy heart and low blood pressure all contribute to reducing the risk of diabetes. Please see Case Study 2.

Obesity increases the risk of osteoarthritis by up to 15 times, says Arthritis Research UK but you can reduce this effect by improving your posture. If you spend a long time doing a particular task, such as being hunched over a laptop or spending excessive amounts of time on your Tablet, Smartphone or similar devices, you could develop poor posture. Balancing your life with moderate running can help to reduce the 'Device hours syndrome', return good posture and give you back some life perspective.

Help You Live Longer

Throughout life, our minds and bodies make a transition and, there may be occasions when we experience creaking joints, slowing metabolism and sluggish memory. But while we can expect our bodies to naturally change over time, running can help reduce or slow the above effects.

There are many studies supporting the fact that runners live longer. One such study by the Stanford University Medical Center (U.S), found that regular runners compared to non-runners had a lower mortality rate. The study was carried out with 500 runners in their 50s and the case was followed for over 20 years - 34% of the non-runners died compared to 15% of the runners in the study.

Improve Bone Density

Bones react to the impact forces of running and as a result become stronger, increasing bone mineral density and so reducing the risk of osteoporosis when we get older. Research confirms that regular running increases bone density more successfully compared to cycling and swimming, as these two sports have low, or no, impact. However, as we will see later, these non-impact sports also have a key role in developing fitness.

Be Good For Your Knees

Many people resist taking up running because they believe it will damage their knees. Well, studies now indicate that running is actually good for the knees. One study at Boston University of Medicine discovered that running stimulated the cartilage in order to repair damage, increasing the production of certain proteins which make the knee stronger. The exceptions to this are people who have had knee surgery or had a serious knee injury. It is also advised that people starting to run who are more than 20lbs (9kg) over weight should return to a safer weight first to avoid over-loading the knee joints.

Enhance Life Style

It is normal to have occasional neck or backache on waking; back stiffness after driving for more than two hours; some aching in the legs after walking for 30 minutes to an hour; needing to move around after an hour of sitting on a hard chair etc. However, it is not normal to have intense pain in one or more joints after carrying shopping; or experiencing difficulty or discomfort getting into a low car or out of a seat. It was mentioned in the abstract that a lot of people (especially the young) are spending many hours per day using their mobile devices, leading to bending over and looking down for long periods. This pattern can also put additional strain on the back and neck muscles.

Having any one of these symptoms is a sign your joints or back are possibly not in their best condition which may have been caused through injury, a sedentary lifestyle or poor posture. Improved fitness can help get your joints moving again and can assist in the reduction of joint pain (especially when coupled with weight control). If in any doubt about your back/joint conditions, please consult a health professional before starting a fitness programme.

Lower the Risk of Diabetes

Consistent aerobic (being able to hold a discussion) exercise like running, in association with a good nutrition plan and weight control, significantly lowers the risk of developing Type 2 diabetes. Running has also been known to reduce or stop the need for medications for people with Type 2 diabetes, using running as an effective means of managing blood glucose.

Reference: U.S. Department of Health and Human Services: "Physical Activity and Health: A Report of the Surgeon General. "American Diabetes Association. Castaneda, C. Diabetes Care, December 2002. Why is this important? - because as at 2015 Diabetes cases have soared by 60%. http://www.bbc.co.uk/news/health-33932930

Reduce the Risk of Cancer

Numerous journals and publications have linked running with a lower risk of cancer. Running can lower the risk of cancers such as those of lung, colon, prostate and liver and, especially breast cancer. Running produces a positive hormonal response and as certain cancers develop from hormonal imbalances your running can help prevent these occurring. According to Cancer Research UK, keeping active could help to prevent around 3,400 cases of cancer every year in the UK.

Boost Immune System
One of the main benefits of running is that it leads to a positive long-term immune response, equipping your body to fight off germs and bacteria. This is why runners generally get fewer colds and infections than more sedentary people.

Reduce Headache and Migraine
Running has been shown to improve blood flow to the brain, reduce muscular tension and to improve hormonal imbalance, all of which are connected to the cause of migraines and frequent headaches. There are rare occurrences of migraines being brought on by running, but on the whole running is beneficial for headache and migraine relief.

Some Case Study examples of how running fitness can benefit your physiology
There are many potential physical benefits of running and, here we share two mini case studies.

Case Study 1 - Cholesterol reduction
You may have heard that exercise is one of the best ways to lower your cholesterol. But how does it work, and what type of exercise is most effective?

The Exercise-Cholesterol Link
Researchers are beginning to have a clearer idea of how exercise lowers cholesterol. "Lots of people, including health professionals like Amit Khera (MD, Director of the University

of Texas), are finding the connections between exercise and cholesterol levels.

One way exercise can help lower cholesterol is by helping you lose - or maintain - weight. Being overweight tends to increase the amount of low-density lipoprotein (LDL) in your blood, the kind of lipoprotein that has been linked to heart disease.

Khera says, "Part of the confusion about the effect of exercise on cholesterol stems from the fact that most early cholesterol studies focused on both exercise and dietary changes, making it hard to tease out which of these factors was actually making the difference. But recent studies have more carefully examined the effect of exercise alone, making it easier to evaluate the relationship between exercise and cholesterol. Researchers now believe there are several mechanisms involved. First, exercise stimulates enzymes that help move LDL from the blood (and blood-vessel walls) to the liver. From there, the cholesterol is converted into bile (for digestion) or excreted. So the more you exercise, the more LDL your body expels.

Secondly, exercise increases the size of the protein particles that carry cholesterol through the blood. Some of those particles are small and dense; some are big and fluffy. "The small, dense particles are more dangerous than the big, fluffy ones because the smaller ones can squeeze into the linings of the heart and blood vessels - and stay there. But now it appears that exercise increases the size of the protein particles that carry both good and bad lipoproteins."

Exactly how much exercise is needed to lower cholesterol has been a matter of some debate. In general, most public health organisations recommend, at a minimum, 20 minutes per day of moderate exercise, such as walking, running, biking or gardening.

In essence, some exercise is better than none and more exercise is better than some.

How Much Will It Help?

Just how much of an effect exercise has on cholesterol is also a matter of debate. Roger Blumenthal (Director of the Ciccarone Preventive Cardiology Center at John Hopkins University), found that the people who benefit the most are those who had the worst diet and exercise habits to begin with. Some of those people, in the study, reduced their LDL by 10-15% and increased their HDL (High Density Lipoprotein) by 20%.

Case Study 2 - Weight Control and Heart Health

One of our fellow runners, whilst not excessively overweight, suffered a heart attack in 2007 and, as part of his rehabilitation, joined a running club. Shortly after recovering from his heart problem, he was able to walk his daughter down the aisle. Frank, 65, who ran through Halifax with the Olympic Torch in 2012 (Figure 1), reckons he is now fitter than ever thanks to taking up running. He has reduced his cholesterol from above 8 to

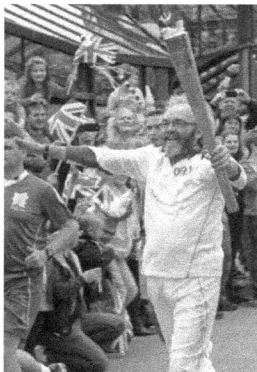

Fig. 1 Frank Chislett with the Olympic Torch. Image by kind permission of Tim Green

around 3 and lost three and a half stone (16kg) in weight.

Frank said: "It sounds bonkers but, for me, having a heart attack has given me a new lease of life. If I hadn't had one I would probably still be the couch potato I was. Not everybody can do what I have done, but I just want to send the message that there can be a great life after a heart attack and the support is terrific."

He has run two marathons and completed several charity runs and is continuing to keep fit and active. To aid his recovery, Frank joined a Cardiac Rehabilitation Unit which was a big help. It is clinically proven that people who attend these programmes have an improved quality of life and live longer than those who don't. For example, the people of Calderdale and Huddersfield have a team of dedicated health professionals running a variety of programmes to help and support heart patients to understand their condition and improve their quality of life.

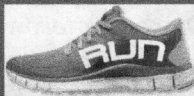

If you haven't been exercising regularly already, it is important to start slowly. Be sure to check with your health professional, so that they can evaluate your current health. This could mean blood pressure or, even a treadmill test to see how your heart reacts when you exercise.

This chapter has concentrated on the physical benefits of running. However, exercise can also improve your emotional situation. In Chapter 2 you will find some valuable information about the emotional benefits that running can bring.

CHAPTER 2

It's All in the Mind

So, what are the emotional benefits of running? We said in the previous chapter that it may come as no surprise that exercise can improve your physical situation. However, you may be pleased to learn that exercise can also bring many mental and emotional benefits. These typically include:

Reducing Stress
Exercise is as good for the mind as it is for the body. Martin and Geoff held highly responsible jobs and found that exercise was an effective way to relax, unwind and solve problems. Running increases serotonin levels in the brain which is good for avoiding stress but also very effective for stress relief. After a busy day, a run works to relieve pressure almost instantly. When you combine running with fresh air and the countryside, your troubles seem less significant.

Improving Memory and Creativity
It really is all in the mind - if you don't use your brain, it wastes away. So, it is important to undertake activities that stimulate it. The more new things you do the better, even if it's just going to a new park. Neurons make new connections when we do something different. Therefore, starting running is a good way to stimulate the brain and to set up new neural pathways.

  Studies have shown* that if you run regularly this can boost your creativity and increase learning capacity. One such study in 2006 at the University of Muenster, Germany, discovered a direct relationship between running and learning ability. So, running can even make you smarter! *Dr Catriona Morrison*

Alleviating Depression and Anxiety

One of the mental benefits of running you hear a lot about is its effect on depression and anxiety. Nowadays many doctors will prescribe running for depression before they prescribe medication due to its continued success. The production of beta endorphins in the brain is the scientific explanation, but there is more to it than that.

Regular exercise has been associated with improved mental well-being and a lower incidence of depression. The Cochrane Review** (the most influential medical review of its kind in the world) has produced a landmark analysis of 23 studies on exercise and depression. One of the major conclusions was that exercise had a 'large clinical impact.'

Have you ever noticed that you feel great after exercise? It turns out that you are not alone, and that exercise may have a big effect on mood and mental well-being. While it might be no surprise that exercise can improve your mood, a good deal of scientific research has been done to discover the possible reasons for this. 'We are what we think' and some researchers argue that exercise may act as a diversion from negative thoughts and could be important in the fight against depression.

There is evidence to indicate that social contact between people who are working out, or involved in sports, may be an important source of satisfaction as well. Still others think that physical activity causes the brain to release chemicals (endorphins) that help us feel good after exercising. Most of the researchers looking at exercise and mood compared groups of people who were exercising to those who were not. They then looked to see if those who were exercising felt better in the short term.

Some researchers compared exercising to more typical treatments for depression such as antidepressant medications or Cognitive Behavioural Therapy. The vast majority of studies have shown that there is a significant association between exercise and improved well-being. Endorphins are natural painkillers and can make us happier. When we are happier and more positive the Dopamine in our brains enters the learning centres making us more receptive to new ideas (Shawn Achor – The Happiness Advantage). This brain stimulation is a great way of keeping us young and enjoying life more.

* Cochrane Reviews are systematic reviews of primary research in human health care and health policy, and are internationally recognised as the highest standard in evidence-based health care. They investigate the effects of interventions for prevention, treatment and rehabilitation. They also assess the accuracy of a diagnostic test for a given condition in a specific patient group and setting. They are published online in The Cochrane Library.

Improving Self-Confidence

Reaching running targets time after time – even small targets – will provide a certain sense of achievement. This will build self-confidence and enhance self-image which spills over into other areas of life, e.g. at work. In other words, achieving running targets lets you believe other obstacles in your life can be overcome with the same mental approach you have towards running fitness.

Helping With Drug Addiction

There are many success stories of people coming off drugs through running - from tobacco and alcohol to the more serious drugs such as Cocaine and Heroin. When someone stops taking drugs there is a hole left in their lives, and running, can conveniently fill this hole – after all, running is something to obsess about!

Case Study – GlasgowGrand Running Team

150 recovering addicts in Glasgow have taken steps to turn their lives around. They did this by forming a running club and entering local races. Addiction often gets lots of bad press but there are many good stories about recovery going on and they don't often get highlighted. However, there are benefits of fitness in dealing with addiction.

This project is related to the Glasgow City Council social work department and links indirectly with the local community addiction team. As well as helping people with alcohol and drug issues they help to move them on into further education, training and employment.

Henry, one of the team members, managed to secure funding for 150 recovering addicts to take part in the Great Scottish Run. Half the money came from the GRAND (Getting Real About Alcohol and Drugs) scheme and the other from Glasgow Life Participants. Named the 'Grand Recovery Runners', all 150 participants ran the Great Scottish Run 10k. Incidentally, at the 2014 event, 40% of the Glasgow Grand running team were female.

The team had joint training sessions in Glasgow Green every Wednesday and all of this was achieved through a

*planning group with representatives from across the city.
Henry is also confident that this run is just the start of things
to come. The response has been very good and Henry
anticipates that more people will want to enter future events.
People are getting better, and getting off drugs, so it's good to
highlight something positive.*

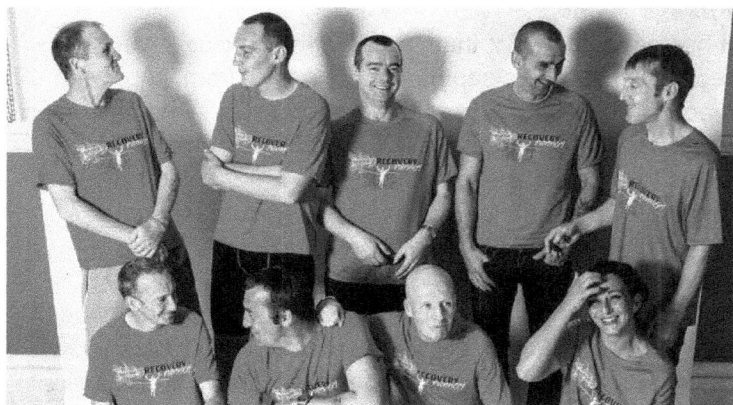

*Fig. 2 Glasgow's Grand recovery Runners. Image by kind permission of Glasgow Grand
Reference: http://news.stv.tv/west-central/
188115-grand-recovery-runners-150-recovering-addicts-to-take-part-in-run/*

Running Helps You Sleep..... and sleep helps you run

In this book, we state that fitness can improve by paying attention to training and diet. However, there's a simple thing that might be overlooked; going to bed earlier. That might help our fitness and, having a regular training regime may also help you to sleep sounder.

Fitness = sleep

It has been shown*** that people who exercise regularly reported that their sleep quality improved, from 'poor' to 'good'. They also reported fewer depressive symptoms, more vitality and less sleepiness in the daytime. As your fitness starts to improve and you adopt a regular training regime, it might be worth noting how your sleep pattern changes.

Sleep = fitness

In David Geier's*** research he showed that getting enough sleep is crucial for athletic performance. His studies show that good sleep can improve speed, accuracy, and reaction time in athletes.

*** David Geier, MD, an orthopedic surgeon and sports medicine specialist in Charleston, SC.

Most people need around eight hours sleep a night. But, if you are in training, you may need more. Just as runners need more calories than most people when they're in training, they need more sleep too. As you are increasing the effort on your body, you may need more time to recover. Not getting enough sleep doesn't only make you tired the next day, it has a big impact on what's happening inside your body, as sleep is the time when your body repairs itself.

One study tracked the Stanford University basketball team for several months. Players added an average of almost two hours sleep a night. The results showed that players increased their speed by 5%, their free throws were 9% more accurate, they had faster reflexes and they felt happier. Other studies have shown similar benefits for football players and other athletes.

Just as with training, getting enough sleep takes commitment. A lot of things can get in the way, like work deadlines, travel arrangements, early morning starts and family commitments but the extra sleep pays off if you can juggle your commitments.

*I*f you have sleeping problems try running earlier in the day. About six hours after a run is the best time to sleep, when the body has cooled down. Try to have a regular schedule. Try and get to bed and get up at the same time every day.

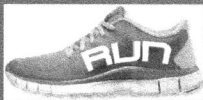

If you have an early start for a race away from home, or a venue you are not familiar with, give yourself plenty of time. This might mean going to bed extra early so that when you arrive at the venue the following day, you will feel fresher and able to make the preparations for your event.

Try to avoid sleep medication, unless a doctor has prescribed it. Studies (*Thornton) show that 'over-the-counter' sleep aids are likely to disturb the quality of your sleep and your performance the next day. It might be better to rely on natural relaxation techniques before bed, such as deep breathing.

It is also advisable to reduce alcohol and caffeine intake, or anything that could disrupt your sleep.

CHAPTER 3

It's a Pain

Introduction

In Chapters 1 and 2 we illustrated how running can bring both physical and emotional benefits. We have seen how exercise might play a part in reducing physical illness, alleviating depression and reducing memory loss. But how can running and other forms of exercise reduce the perception of pain and therefore help us to manage our lives better?

Athletes and pain experts agree that prolonged exercise raises people's spirits. Many believe that the body's own opioids, or more commonly known as endorphins, are the cause of this. More recently this has been proven by the use of MRI scanning of the brain. Researchers at *TU München and the University of Bonn** demonstrated the existence of an 'endorphin-driven feel-good factor'. In an imaging study they were able to show increased release of endorphins in certain areas of runners' brains during a two-hour exercise session. These results may also be relevant for patients suffering from chronic pain, because the body's own endorphins are produced in areas of the brain which are involved in the suppression of pain.

Runner's High – reducing the perception of pain

Sports have long been seen as being responsible for: reducing stress, relieving anxiety, enhancing mood and decreasing the perception of pain. The 'endorphin-driven feel-good factor' that accompanies running even led to the creation of its own term, **'Runner's High'**.

Endorphins facilitate the body's own pain suppression by influencing the way the body passes on pain and processes it in the nervous system and brain. The increased production of endorphins resulting from running could also serve as the body's own pain-killer, which is a potent potential therapeutic option.

The scientific background

This section gives an overview of some scientific knowledge about what exercise really does to our bodies and our brains. Most of us are aware of what happens to the body when we exercise. We build more muscle or more stamina and we feel how daily activities like climbing stairs become easier if we exercise regularly. When it comes to our brain and mood though, the connection isn't so easy to describe. So, what triggers happiness, mood and pain suppression in our brains when we exercise?

If you start exercising, your brain recognises this as a moment of stress. As your blood pressure increases, your brain thinks you are either fighting the enemy or fleeing from it (The so called flight or fight syndrome). To protect yourself and your brain from stress, a protein called BDNF is released (Brain-Derived Neurotrophic Factor). BDNF adds a protective and also reparative element to your memory neurons.

That's why we often feel so at ease and why things are clear after exercising and eventually why we are happier after a run. Sometimes before we exercise we carry the burden of the world on our shoulders; we may have worries about work or family, or we may not be able to solve a puzzling problem.

These tasks, which seemed difficult to resolve, are given a new perspective and seem easier to tackle after exercise.

At the same time as BDNF is released, endorphins are also are released in your brain. According to McGovern** this is the main purpose of your endorphins. As seen earlier, endorphins tend to minimise the discomfort of exercise, block the feeling of pain and are even associated with a feeling of euphoria. Overall, there is a lot going on inside our brain and it is a lot more active during exercise than when we are just sitting down or actually concentrating mentally (Hillman ***).

Figure 3 illustrates an MRI scan showing increased brain activity during exercise. This shows a composite of 20 students' brains engaged in a test. The image on the left is taken after the students sat quietly, the image on the right is taken after 20 minutes walking.

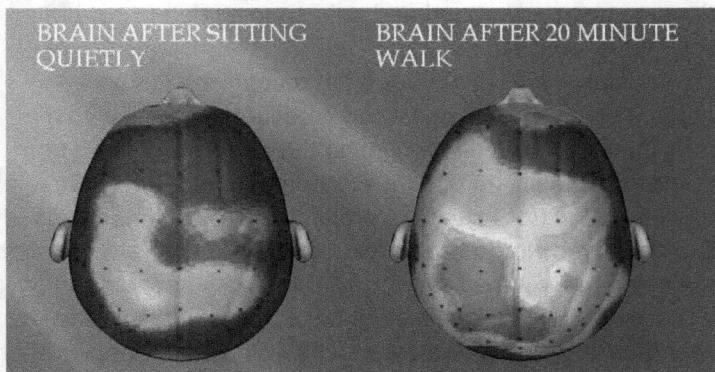

BRAIN AFTER SITTING QUIETLY

BRAIN AFTER 20 MINUTE WALK

Fig. 3 MRI scan showing increased brain activity during exercise.
Reproduced by kind permission of Dr. Chuck Hillman, University of Illinois.

So, BDNF and endorphins are the reasons exercise makes us feel so good. Interestingly, they have a very similar and addictive behaviour like that of Morphine, Heroine or Nicotine. The only difference is that exercise is, actually, **good** for us. Please also refer to Chapter 2 where we gave the example of the 150 recovering substance misuse addicts, in Glasgow. These addicts have taken the steps to turn their lives around by starting jogging, forming a running club and entering local races.

Sustainability

We have explored the basic foundations of why, and how, exercising makes us happy and what happens inside our brain (a little insight into the scientific aspect). It is now important to see how we can trigger this in an optimal and longer lasting way.

The increase of the BDNF proteins in our brain acts as a mood enhancer and the effects are similar to drug addiction, as we have just mentioned. So when you start exercising, the feeling of euphoria is the highest: "The release of endorphins has this addictive effect, and more exercise is, therefore, needed to achieve the same level of euphoria over time." **. This means that if you have never exercised before, or not for a long time, your happiness gains will be the highest if you start **now**!

Knowing how much exercise to do to help relieve pain

During our lifetime, we may develop postural imbalances; for example, from carrying a child on one hip or habitually carrying a bag on one shoulder. These imbalances or other factors such as: cancer, shingles, arthritis, ageing or injury can trigger pain in the back, hips, knees, ankles, shoulders and other parts of the body. If you do feel **chronic** pain (pain that has lasted more than 12 weeks, as opposed to acute pain that is a sensation to alert us to possible injury), it is probably taking a toll on your quality of life and, it is important to recognise just how far exercise and fitness might be able to contribute to alleviating your symptoms.

If you have back or joint pain, there are probably some times when all you want to do is lie in bed all day. We understand that this is tempting, but it might actually make your problem worse. Ignoring the pain will not make it go away completely. Neither will avoiding all motions that trigger discomfort. In fact, limiting your range of movement can lead to weaker muscles which may compound joint trouble. This could affect your posture and create a further set of complications. Whilst pain relief medication and cold/hot packs may offer some relief, these may only be temporary fixes.

Health Professionals used to prescribe bed rest for back pain and other chronic pain conditions, but studies by Nessler **** have found that people who exercise and stay flexible manage their pain much better than those who don't. Trent Nessler, Vice President of Champion Sports Medicine in Birmingham, USA says that "Exercise improves your pain threshold, especially when coupled with cardiovascular, strengthening, and flexibility exercise".

The right set of exercises can be a long-lasting way to manage joint pain. When practiced regularly, joint pain relief workouts might permit you to postpone, or even avoid, surgery on a problematic joint that has been troubling you for years, by strengthening key supportive muscles and restoring flexibility. Over time, you may find limitations that you had learned to live with will begin to ease. Tasks and fun-filled life opportunities that have been passing you by may come back into reach, too.

Getting Started

If you do have a chronic pain condition like back, hip, knee, or shoulder problem, you should not begin an exercise programme without guidance. We strongly advise that you check with your Health Professional (Doctor) first, and then seek an expert to help you develop a tailored exercise programme just for you. You could ask a physiotherapist or athletic trainer to show you what exercises are appropriate, given your condition. These exercise specialists may conduct a postural assessment to see how you stand and how you walk.

Beyond the benefits to your joints, becoming more active can help you stay independent long into your later years and regular activity is good for your heart and sharpens the mind. It reduces blood pressure, enhances morale, eases stress and helps control weight. Exercise improves your balance and could make falls less likely. Improving your range of movement may also support longevity and all of this can be achieved at a comfortable pace and very low cost.

Case Study - How exercise affects nerve pain - Fibromyalgia

Here we present a short case study to demonstrate how

running and fitness can alleviate pain. In this example, we look at the common complaint, Fibromyalgia, but other painful conditions can also be improved through running.

Fibromyalgia syndrome is a disorder that affects the muscles and soft tissues of the body. It is believed that fibromyalgia intensifies painful sensations by affecting the way that the brain processes pain signals. A significant body of research shows that, for people with fibromyalgia, exercise can improve their physical and emotional well-being, prevent the muscle wasting that avoiding activity can bring, and for some even alleviate pain. Fibromyalgia sufferers often become less and less active as the pain takes over, scared to make any kind of movement that could increase the pain. That starts a vicious, debilitating circle.

This fear, which is seen to varying degrees among people with fibromyalgia, is a huge obstacle to getting people to be more physically active, and research***** shows that walking, strength training, and even stretching can improve physical pain and emotional well-being in fibromyalgia patients.

One patient finds relief through movement

*This patient, said her pain, which intensified around age 30, was 'excruciating'. On a scale of 1 to 10, she would tell her pain doctor, 'it's 20'. Before fibromyalgia, this lady of 50 years of age, was an active woman who loved running and cycling. After the Fibromyalgia syndrome developed, her day-to-day pain levels became more of a 'roller coaster' with unpredictable swelling. But in the 20 years since the pain began, she has found exercise to be one of the **critical tools** in managing her neck and shoulder pain. "Exercise is* number 1 for me," she explained. This woman mostly does cardiovascular work and then weights. Her routine includes cycling, running and walking and, as she gets older, anything which conditions her muscles seems to help.

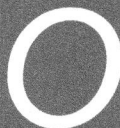

*O*ver the years, Martin and Geoff have found that running is made up of a number of factors; training, diet, preparation etc. However, there have been times when the onset of pain, during a phase of a race, would normally force runners to stop. The Authors recognised that the perception of pain can be alleviated by focusing on a specific thought to get you through that phase of the race i.e. thinking of the pizza at the finish line!

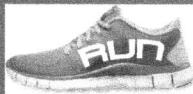

* University of Bonn. "Runners' High Demonstrated: Brain Imaging Shows Release Of Endorphins In Brain." ScienceDaily. ScienceDaily, 6 March 2008.

** Dr. Mark McGovern , Associate Professor of Psychiatry and of Community and Family Medicine at Dartmouth Medical School, New Hampshire, USA.The Effects of exercise on the Brain. http://serendip.brynmawr.edu/bb/neuro/neuro05/web2/mmcgovern.html

*** 20 minutes of exercise boosts test performance, Dr Chuck Hillman, University of Illinois.

**** Trent Nessler, PT, DPT, MPT, Vice President, Champion Sports Medicine, Birmingham, Alabama, Exercise and Pain relief.

*****Dr.Daniel Rooks, Assistant Professor of Medicine at Harvard Medical School.

CHAPTER 4

Let's Get Started

The first 20 or so minutes of moving around, if someone has been really sedentary, can provide most of the health benefits. You can get prolonged life and reduced disease risk - all in the first 20 minutes of being active. So really, you can relax and don't have to be on the look-out for the next killer work-out. All you have to do is get some focused, 20 minutes in to get the full happiness boost every day.

Sometimes, even when the authors, Martin and Geoff are busy they make time to fit in a short exercise session (a 20-minute run or a few miles on the turbo trainer) as they know this will make them feel better. Research shows that on exercise days, people's moods significantly improved after exercising.

The important thing is to make your exercise and running lots of fun, so let's **get started**:

- If you wish to run in the morning, put your running kit over your alarm clock or phone when you go to bed: This technique sounds rather simple, but is one of the most powerful ones. If you put everything the way you want it for your morning run, before you go to sleep, you will have a much easier time to convince yourself to put your kit on the following morning.

- Track your exercises and log them at the same time after every exercise: When exercising regularly, it will become a habit. One way to achieve this is to create a so called 'reward', that will remind you of the good feelings you get from exercising. Web applications or fitness apps might be handy. You might wish to try out 'RunKeeper' to log your work-outs or just keep a written diary. You can refer to the Appendix for more information on how technology (Apps etc) may help. It's good to have a very clear logging process in place. Try to log your work-out just before you go into the shower or when you walk back into your home after a run.

- You might want to think about starting small and then start even smaller: Here is a little secret. When you first start exercising, do it for five minutes per day, three times a week. Can you imagine that? 'That's nothing' you might be thinking and you are right, because the task is so easy and anyone can succeed with it. You can really start to make a habit out of it. Try no more than five or 10 minutes if you are getting started then build to the 20 minute target and beyond.

Start by lots of walking, burn off the weight, then start a 'walk-run' programme. Try the 'lamppost approach' where you walk and run, alternately, between the lampposts on a road. As you become more comfortable you can jog for two lamppost lengths and walk one. You can then increase accordingly until you can run your intended distance.

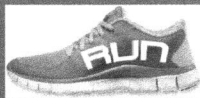

How easy is it to start running?

There are not many activities which give such enormous benefits and are as easy to take up as running. Alright, you could start playing Tiddly Winks but, whilst that is a very pleasant pastime, it is unlikely to bring you the physical, emotional and psychological benefits of running - we don't know of a Tiddly Winks High! You can start running inside your house, around and close to your home or even in a nearby leafy park just to get started. Nobody will be putting any pressure on you to be an Olympic Athlete and you are better off running just very short distances to start with. You can go running at any time of the day or night, to suit your preferences and circumstances. There is no longer a stigma to people running the streets, so go out there and enjoy! You may even find that you gain respect from others.

What would you like to achieve from exploring and starting running?

Whenever we take up something new it is always useful to have some kind of goal so that we can measure ourselves against what we intended to achieve.

What are your reasons for wanting to consider running? Could it be a sport, hobby, conduit for meeting people, stopping smoking, controlling weight or just getting a little bit fitter and healthier?

Where are you now?

On a scale of 0 to 10, where are you today? Why not complete the wheel shown in Figure 4 to see where you might want to place your emphasis. *If you do not like scribbling in your book then we have included a copy of this wheel at the back of the book.*

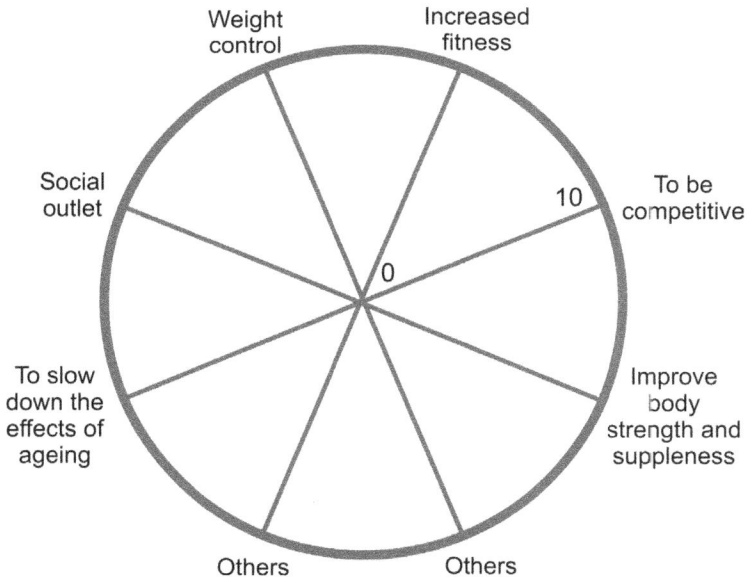

Figure 4 Running Goals Wheel

As you will see, each segment is labelled to represent possible beneficial effects from running. With **0** in the centre and **10** on the outside edge of the circle, rate your current level of satisfaction for each area by making a mark along each of the lines. There are a couple of 'others' or blank areas where you can add your own categories. You may even wish to select one from the cloud inside the front cover of this book.

Then, look at the circle and ask: 'if I have to select one area on which to focus, which would it be in terms of giving me the highest impact or biggest benefit from running? You don't have to pick the category with the lowest score. For the selected category alone, clearly identify what '10' will be like (when you are satisfied with improvements here). This is your

Inspirational Running Goal...

...Lets Get Started!

There are lots more great ideas for how you can get into the habit of running. We are sure that if you dedicate just very little time, you can get into a useful exercise routine that makes you happier, more productive and more relaxed than ever before.

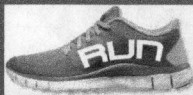

CHAPTER 5

You Wear it Well

Running Kit - What do you need?

Unlike golf or other popular pastimes, running requires only very simple clothing and accessories. The main cost items are the shoes which we will look at in more detail in this chapter.

To go running you just need to have suitable comfortable clothes that will keep you cool in the summer (Figure 5) and warm in the winter (Figure 6). Basic running kit would comprise: a pair of mid-priced shoes, a few tops (long and short sleeved), a pair of shorts, a pair of long bottoms (known as Tracksters), a sweatshirt, and a waterproof/windproof jacket. Add to this, a hat and a pair of gloves and you are kitted out for most weather conditions. It is also advisable, if running outside at dusk or in the dark, to acquire a high visibility jacket (or bib) and flashing torch and armbands.

To get started it is important not to become obsessed with the latest fad and this year's colour. Instead, look at offers for last year's kit (very often the difference is only colour). Make sure that whatever you buy is comfortable and will hopefully do the job you require. Avoid kit that is too tight, as movement is very important. Also, you may need to carry a water-resistant top if rain is likely, so small and lightweight is the order of the day.

As you become more used to running, you may wish to try kit from the vast range of Technical Wear that is widely available. The advantages of these garments are comfort and lightness. They wash and dry very quickly and when wet are less heavy than cotton. One limitation of cotton is that when wet, either from rain or perspiration, it can become heavy and uncomfortable. Cotton based kit can however be useful after a race or training run for its softness and warmth i.e. this is where a sweatshirt comes into its own.

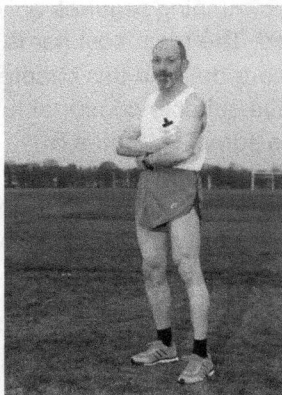

Fig. 5 Summer Kit   *Fig. 6 Winter Kit*

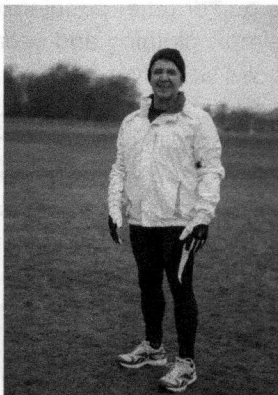

Equally if you want an occasional treat, you could buy the latest piece of kit especially when you have attained a personal target. It is always worth visiting web sites specialising in sports kit e.g. www.wiggle.co.uk or www. northernrunner.com (In the References section, towards the back of the book, we have listed some popular running stores). It is also worth looking at the shop that might be supporting a race you are doing, as they often have a stall with good offers available. If you are a club member you may also be able to benefit from a club discount with your local running store.

Sun protection

Why is this important? – There is an increase in the number of cases of skin cancer around the world and in the UK alone there are around 100,000 people diagnosed with skin cancer each year. Skin cancers are caused by damage from the sun's ultraviolet (UV) rays. Therefore, it is sensible to consider taking protective measures against the sun in order to reduce the risk of skin disease and to help you enjoy your outdoor pursuits.

Sun cream – We recommend that you select a cream that you are familiar with and one that suits your skin type. If unsure, ask your local pharmacist to recommend a type of cream for you.

Protecting your eyes – One, often overlooked, aspect of sun protection is that of the eyes. Even on a non-sunny day, the light intensity carries damaging UV rays. Therefore, we recommend wearing a pair of appropriate sunglasses. Not all sunglasses offer the required protection, so when you are selecting a pair, consider the following requirements:

- The CE Mark and British Standard (BS EN 1836:2005)
- A UV 400 label
- A statement that the sunglasses offer 100% UV protection

Also, we encourage you to think about the sides of your eyes, and consider sunglasses with wide or wraparound arms.

Shoes

The most important piece of kit to get right is your **shoes**.
Some experimentation may be needed and consideration
needs to be given to the type of terrain you will initially train/
race on. As time goes by you may find that your range of
footwear will grow as you run on a mixture of surfaces i.e.
road, trails, fells or maybe track. Take advice from shoe
specialists who often have a running machine in store
to analyse your gait and match a shoe to you. Also give
consideration to the colour you choose; light colours look
good in the spring/summer but in winter a darker colour may
be better. See Figure 7, Shoe Anatomy

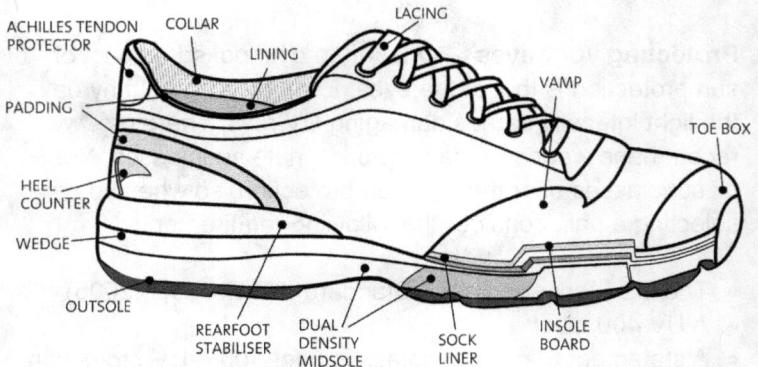

Figure 7, Shoe Anatomy

Which shoe type for you?

Running shoes come in many shapes and sizes. Shoes are based on the design of the human foot and interestingly the human foot also comes in many shapes and sizes. To help you find the right shoe, you could try the simple 'bathroom floor' test.

This test works by leaving a shape of your wet footprint on the bathroom floor. When you get out of the shower or bath and step on to the floor, you will notice that it leaves a wet foot mark. Whilst this is not an exact science, it is a good indicator of your foot type. There are basically three recognised foot types; Normal Arch, Low Arch and High Arch (also known respectively as Neutral, Pronation and Supination) as shown in Figure 8. Having this knowledge may help you when you go to buy your first pair of running shoes.

We would also advise that you go to a specialist running store to get a more detailed view of your overall running style/gait.

	Foot Type (Arch)	Alignment	Recommended Shoe Type
Neutral	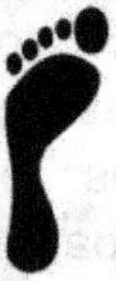 Normal Arch	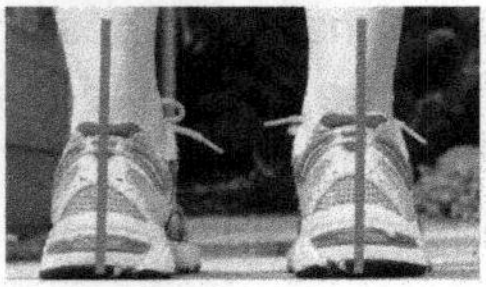	Cushioned, Neutral shoe
Pronation	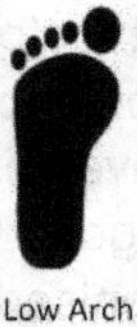 Low Arch	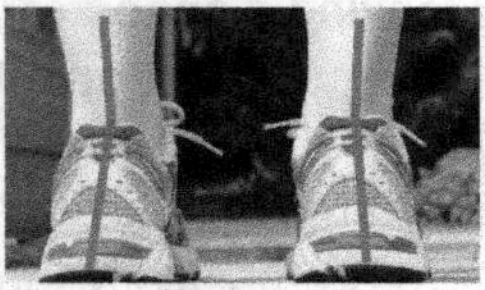	Supportive stability shoe with firm midsole
Supination	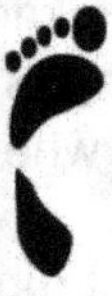 High Arch	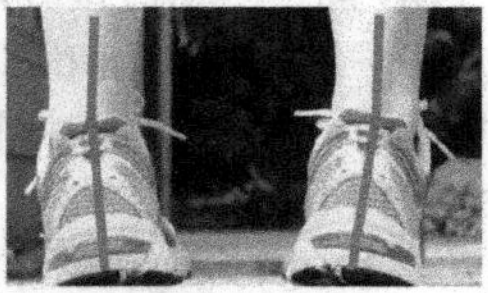	Highly cushioned shoe with less arch support

Fig. 8 Foot Types

Fit

Having looked at the different foot types, you may need to try a variety of brands and styles to find the perfect fit for you. Each shoe brand and model will have a slightly different shape, contour, forefoot width and heel width. The following list is an indicator for a good fit.

Shape - The shape of feet vary. Some feet are relatively straight and others are slightly curved. When selecting a pair of shoes, it is best to take a look at all the running shoes and look for the general shape that matches your foot type (higher arched feet are more curved, whereas neutral feet are straighter).   Matching the shoe shape to your foot is perhaps the most important part of selecting the right running shoe. Be patient and try on several different models.

Forefoot width - Some people are more comfortable with a snug fit while others prefer a little 'toe wiggle' room.

Length – When you stand with the shoes laced up, there should be a finger's width gap between the longest toe and the end of the shoe.

Heel cup – Heels also vary in their width so you will need to try on different shoes to find the brand or model that cradles your heel snuggly.

Sole
As mentioned above, you need to select the right sole for the terrain on which you will be running. Typically sole configurations, as shown in Figure 9, include:

Waffle (for Fell running)
Trail (for a mixture of road and country trails)
Spike (for Track and Cross Country)
Road (for Tarmac)
Racing flat (for Road Racing)

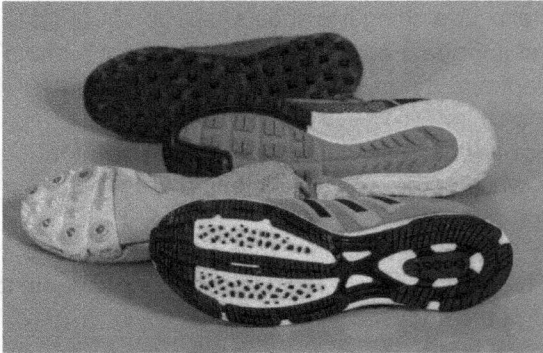

Fig. 9 Running shoe configurations

Further points to consider

- Selecting a shoe that matches your foot type and provides you with a perfect fit is more important than the technological features. Try not to be persuaded by the latest fashion or feature.
- For a running shoe to recover from a run they require about 24 hours. It is best not to wear your training shoes when you are not training. If feasible, try to have at least two pairs of training shoes. This helps a running shoe to recover from a run and, it gives your biomechanics some variety.
- It is good practice to replace your shoes regularly. Runners training regularly in a pair of shoes for, say, more than four months are more likely to be injured as a result of shoe deterioration. If you are beginning to feel more aches and pains, it is advisable to consider how much use

your shoes have had. Unfortunately, it is impossible to predict how much training a shoe will be able to sustain and still offer you the support and cushioning you need.

Using this knowledge will help you when you select your next pair of shoes.

onsider a lightweight trainer for the road with a little cushioning and a similar off road version with a chunkier sole for greater grip. Be aware that some of the bulky trainers can be heavier. Always double-knot your laces! It is also useful (if funds allow) to have more than one pair of trainers on the go to allow your feet to assume subtly different positions. This may help with long-term injury prevention or even relieving tiredness in your legs.
...Martin once ran the Northern Cross Country race in a pair of spikes. On lap 2 they totally disintegrated so he ran the last two laps in his socks – This was most embarrassing and, the moral of the story is to check your kit before you run.

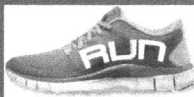

Compression Wear
As you begin to increase your mileage, you may benefit from wearing compression garments. Compression wear is close-fitting clothing - from socks to base layers and shirts. These garments contain high Lycra content (or similar elasticated materials) that squeezes and hugs the muscles that are important in efficient running. This type of kit may help you

train more efficiently, avoid common injuries and recover quicker.

Compression garments have previously been used in clinical settings for treating conditions such as deep vein thrombosis (DVT). Studies have reported positive results in the effectiveness of compression wear to help improve deep venous velocity, venous return, and help to reduce venous pooling in diseased, post operative, inactive hospitalised patients. More recently, these garments have been adopted by beginners and serious athletes alike.

Compression Tops
Compression tops provide core support around your stomach, sides and lower back, which can become fatigued - particularly on long runs. Tops train the breathing by gently squeezing and supporting the chest on each inhalation. This encourages a more focused breathing style and may even reduce the risk of a painful stitch. A compression top can deliver support for the back, giving a more upright approach to your run. Better posture and improved breathing should lead to improved running.

Compression Tights and Compression Socks
These can rapidly reduce recovery time and minimise delayed onset muscle soreness (DOMS). They can also reduce muscle oscillation, particularly through the quadriceps and calf. Lactic acid is flushed out by the squeezing of muscles and increases venous return - which may help reduce cramping.

Compression socks, as well as increasing venous return,

help deliver oxygen to muscles with a tight fit around the foot and a graduated squeeze up the calf. Figure 10.

Some researchers say that compression socks do not have any major physiological influences but runners usually state that wearing them results in improved performance, reduced calf strain, faster recovery times and reduced perceived muscle soreness.

Fig. 10 Geoff wearing Compression Socks, even in the summer.

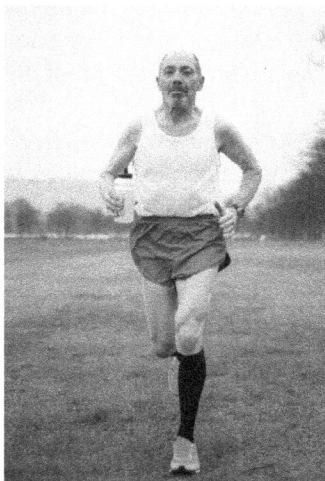

The Science
Blood Lactate - or lactic acid is a by-product of specific exercise regimes and raised levels can lead to fatigued muscles and a reduction in running performance.

Venous Return – this is often abbreviated to VR, and refers to the flow of blood back to the heart.

Muscle Oscillation – is the natural vibration that occurs as a muscle is flexed, or it experiences impact from the ground. This is often seen as a slow motion rippling movement up your leg as your foot hits the ground.

Delayed Onset Muscle Soreness (DOMS) - Describes the

general stiffness you feel between 24 and 72 hours following strenuous exercise. DOMS is the result of over-exercised muscles.

Exercise Induced Muscle Damage (EIMD) - This is a general term, used by some sports scientists, to describe the muscular wear and tear caused through exercise.

Graduated Compression - To improve blood flow, some compression wear varies the amount of squeeze along its length. For example, compression socks often have graduations from the ankle up to the top of the calf.

Sizing guide

When you go to buy Compression Wear, you will be guided to measure your respective body area and use a sizing guide to determine the optimum fit for you. It might appear that you are guided to buy a 'size too small' but, usually, the guides are right. Martin bought some new compression socks, over the internet, for his Triathlons and they fit perfectly.

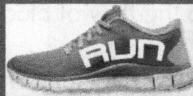

*P*aula Radcliffe set a women's Marathon world record of 2:15:25 in 2003, whilst wearing compression socks. During the 2014 UK IRONMAN Triathlon, Martin also wore compression socks and, whilst his Marathon time was not as good as Paula's he did meet the race cut off times, and his calf muscles were in good condition afterwards.

CHAPTER 6

Keeping Safe and Healthy

The Medical Angle

As we have seen, generally speaking, exercise brings with it very positive benefits. However, here we would like to reiterate that before you start running it is advisable to visit your GP in order to have a basic medical check.

Being seen and being in the right places

In some countries you don't have that many sunny days and, sometimes you may need to go running at night (or in the morning) when the lighting is poor. For example, if you are looking after children, or working during the day and your only opportunity is to run in the evening. On these occasions, it is essential that you make sure you are visible to other road users. Being seen in the dark can be easily achieved by wearing high visibility clothing (as described earlier) and shown in Figure 11. Also, at a very small cost, you can buy flashing armbands from a number of superstores or sports outlets. These accessories allow you to go out and run in the dusk or dark with increased confidence.

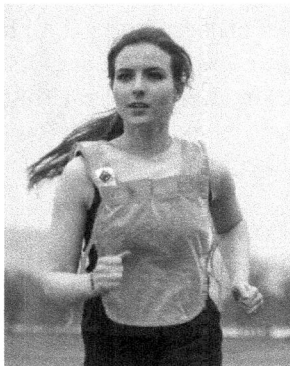

Fig. 11 High Visibility Bib

Safety with/around children

Running with groups of young children can also be good fun. Just make sure they are old enough to jog along with you. Ensure they are wearing suitable kit and have warmed up properly. If running in poor light ensure the children (and you) wear high visibility clothing.

It is OK for you to take your toddler for a little jog but, please be aware that children are not just small adults and there may be particular considerations around bone development.

Bone development - The skeleton of a child is mostly cartilage, which is softer than bone and can bend more easily. The process by which cartilage becomes bone begins very early in life in special growth areas in the bones, called growth plates. These growth plates are the weakest part of the bone and can be easily injured by a sudden force or a repeated force. The good news is that mild forces, encountered during jogging, can stimulate bone growth, but it is best for a child to avoid excessive forces when they are growing.

UK Athletics recommends the following running distances for children and young teens: Under 9s maximum - 1.5km (around 1 mile), under 11s - 1.5km to 2.5km and under 13s - 3km to 5km. Most UK Athletics clubs have a minimum joining age of eight years. You could contact your local running club to confirm this.

Be with others – fitness is a social thing!
Fitness Clubs and other groups

When you start exercising you may feel self-conscious about being seen out on your own, but don't be put off. You are the one receiving the benefits of running, or other activities.

To help cope with the feeling of being on your own you could join a club. Training with other like-minded people who will have, or who are experiencing, the beginning of a new journey can be mentally stimulating and highly beneficial for your general health.

Most clubs, e.g. running clubs, have groups at many levels from *beginner* through *improver* to *advanced* and *elite* so there should be a group to suit you. Meeting other people helps you to develop your fitness and then you may wish to progress to competitive running. So, you can 'run for fun', 'cycle for fun' or 'achieve specific goals'.

For information on running clubs and races, please check out:

UK: http://www.britishathletics.org.uk/grassroots/search/

Europe: http://www.runinternational.eu/ or https://www.mynextrun.com/

USA: http://www.runningintheusa.com/

Planning a running route

Whether you are on your own, or with a group, these are some of the items you should consider for your session:

Distance – determine the ideal/maximum distance you wish to cover and think about 'get home contingencies' if you get tired, ill or injured. i.e. can you get a bus or a taxi home?

Route – determine if you wish to complete a circular route, an out-and-back route or multi-loops.

Mixed ability – If you have a mixed ability group and some of the runners can only run say one third of the target distance, then plan a three lap route to please all abilities.

Terrain – Depending on your interest or forthcoming event, choose a terrain to match. E.g., if you are training for a Marathon, you may wish to run on the Canal Towpath.

Ascent/descent – Depending on your ability (and that of the group) select hills with the ideal gradient. In the early days of running, don't try to tackle very steep hills as this might be difficult and could put you off running. Similarly, running downhill can also be quite challenging and may take a little bit of getting used to.

Traffic – Wherever possible avoid routes with heavy traffic.

Planning aids – By all means, use your local knowledge or, even an OS Map to determine your route. However, you can also use one of the many internet-based route planning tools. i.e. MapMyRun.

Carrying out a risk assessment
It is advisable and responsible, whether running alone or with a group, to carry out a risk assessment. This does not have to be complicated or onerous but should contain the following as a minimum:

Route - Plan the route for your session, as above.

Clothing - Ensure you have the correct clothing, footwear and visibility for the duration of the session.

Group - Know the number of people in your group and be aware of any particular existing conditions; such as impaired vision, Epilepsy, Asthma etc.

Cover – If you have a large group (say more than 10) it is useful to nominate someone to stay at the back of the group.

Emergencies - Have an emergency plan to cater for ill or injured runners.

Contact details – It is useful to have a charged mobile phone with contact numbers for the local hospital and someone, back at base, who can support as required.

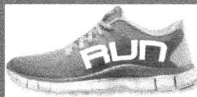

efore running, check the basics: tie your shoelaces correctly, make sure you are visible, know your route and let someone, back at base, know your run route.

CHAPTER 7

Training and Injury Prevention

Introduction

So far in this book, we have explored the fundamentals of running and fitness, and outlined the associated physical and emotional benefits. We also talked a little about running kit and safety in order to get you going. In this Chapter we concentrate on the next phase of your journey by looking at the four steps to fitness, which includes **suppleness & flexibility**, **stretching**, **strengthening** exercises and **fitness training**. After this we help you to understand how and why injuries may occur but, more importantly, we provide some useful tips on how to prevent and manage injuries.

The Four Steps to Fitness

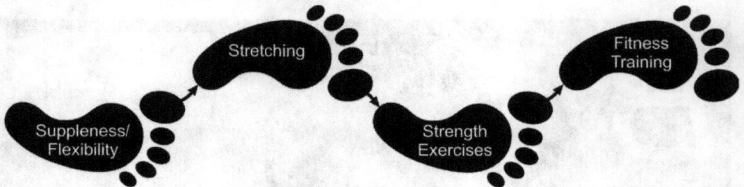

Suppleness/Flexibility → Stretching → Strength Exercises → Fitness Training

Principal Muscle Groups used in Running

Before we start looking at flexibility and stretching we thought it would be a good idea to show you the key muscle groups that you might use in your fitness regime.
These are shown in Figure 12a and 12b:

You may be in reasonably good health or, you may have limited mobility. This could be because of a chronic illness or condition, stiff joints, an injury, lack of exercise or stubborn weight issues. Whatever your situation, you can take some significant steps towards improving your general fitness and reaping the benefits this brings (as outlined in Chapters 1 and 2).

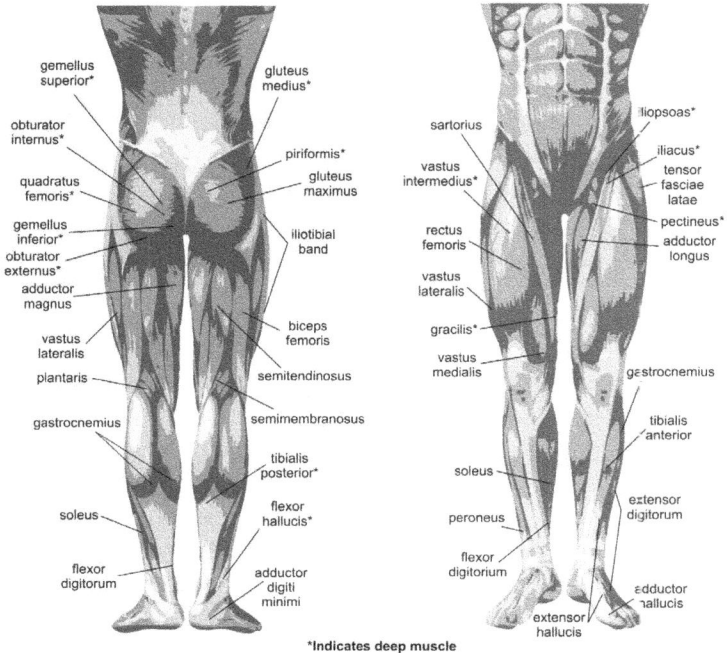

*Indicates deep muscle

Fig. 12a and 12b Lower body Anatomy (Back and Front).

Of course, if you do have a mobility condition, as each one is different, **we recommend that you talk to your Health professional before embarking on a fitness programme**. This section discusses ways in which you can, even with limited mobility, create a workout that suits your needs and improves your situation. We will show you some basic physical movements that you can do with your upper body, lower body, or both.

he exercises illustrated in this chapter can also be helpful in increasing the suppleness of all people starting to get fit, whether you have limited movement or not.

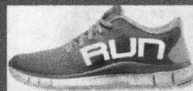

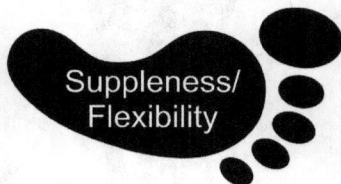

Suppleness/ Flexibility

Home flexibility exercises
These home exercises are ideal if you are not very active but want to improve your health, lift your mood and remain independent. Don't worry if you haven't done much for a while as these exercises are easy, gentle and can be done indoors.

The following exercises can also be carried out in a SITTING or STANDING position. For the chair-based exercises, choose a chair that is stable, solid and without wheels. You should be able to sit with your feet flat on the floor and knees bent at right angles. Avoid chairs with arms, as this will restrict your movement. Build up slowly and aim to gradually increase the repetitions of each exercise over time. Try to do these exercises at least twice a week and combine them with the other routines to help improve strength, balance and co-ordination.

Chair exercises effectively assist relatively immobile individuals, or anyone recovering from injury, to exercise and move without putting undue pressure or strain on their bodies. Movement works to lubricate joints and keep them flexible, strengthen and stabilise individual muscles and increase blood circulation. These exercise and movement outcomes, if you are relatively immobile, result in a decreased number of falls and an increased ability to better accomplish day-to-day physical activities. Unless otherwise stated, it is best to perform these exercises on a straight-backed chair with your feet firmly on the ground.

Chest stretch

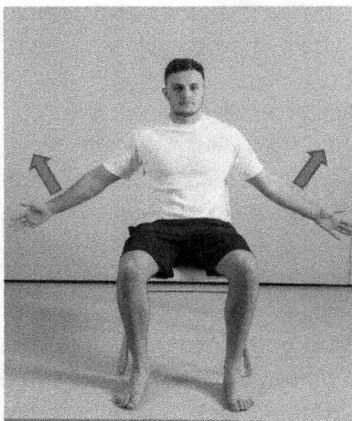 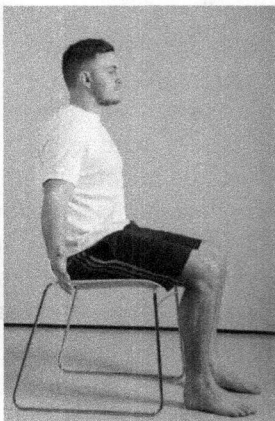

Fig. 13a   *Fig. 13b*

This stretch is good for posture.
Sit upright and away from the back of the chair. Pull your shoulders back and down. Extend your arms out to the side. Figure 13a.

Gently push your chest forwards and up until you feel a stretch across your chest.

Hold for 5 to 10 seconds and repeat five times. Figure 13b.

Upper body twist

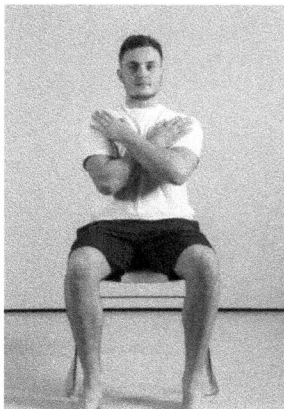 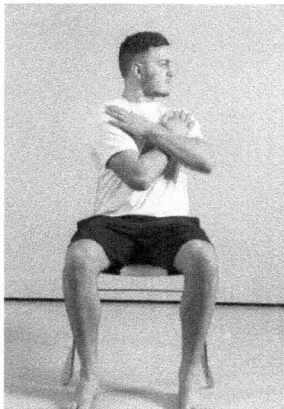

Fig. 14a   *Fig. 14b*

This stretch will develop and maintain flexibility in the upper back.

Sit upright with your feet flat on the floor, cross your arms and reach for your shoulders. Figure 14a.

Without moving your hips, turn your upper body to the left as far as is comfortable. Hold for 5 seconds. Figure 14b.

Repeat on the right side. Do five on each side.

Hip marching

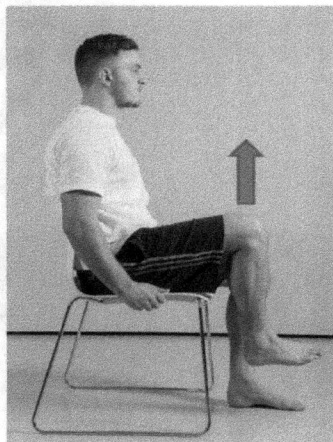

Fig. 15

This exercise will strengthen hips and thighs and improve flexibility.
Sit upright and do not lean on the back of the chair. Hold on to the sides of the chair.
Lift your right leg slowly with your knee bent as far as is comfortable. Place your foot down with control. Figure 15.
Repeat with the opposite leg.
Do five lifts with each leg..

Ankle stretch

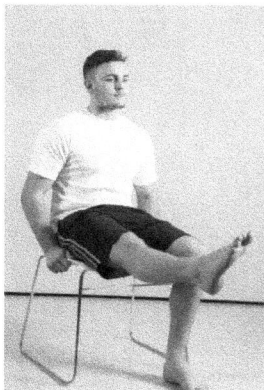 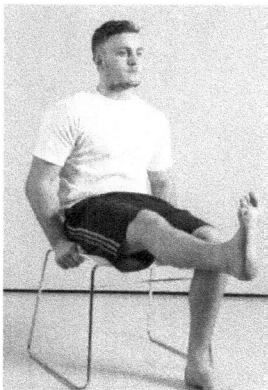

Fig. 16a   *Fig.16b*

This stretch will improve ankle flexibility.
Sit upright, hold on to the side of the chair and straighten your right leg with your foot off the floor.
With your leg straight and raised, point your toes away from you. Figure 16a.
Point your toes back towards you. Figure 16b.
Try two sets of five stretches with each foot.

Arm raises

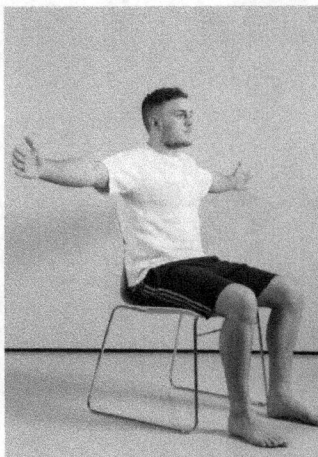 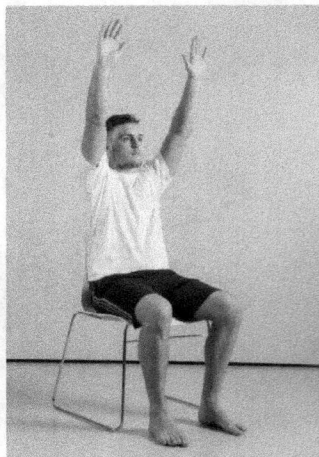

Fig. 17a   *Fig. 17b*

This exercise builds shoulder strength.
Sit upright with your arms by your sides.
With palms forwards, raise both arms out and to the side
(Figure 17a) and up as far as is comfortable (Figure 17b).
Return to the starting position.
Keep your shoulders down and arms straight throughout.
Breathe out as you raise your arms and breathe in as you
lower them. Repeat five times.

Neck rotation

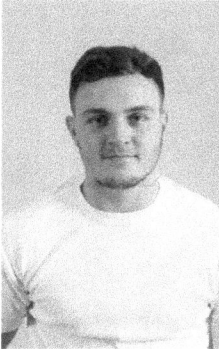 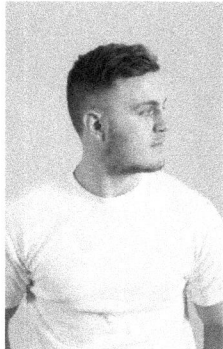 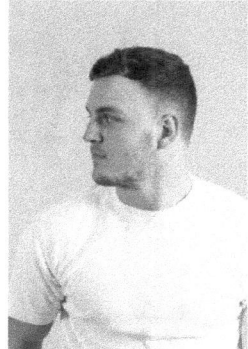

Fig. 18a   *Fig. 18b*   *Fig. 18c*

This stretch is good for improving neck mobility and flexibility.

Sit upright with your shoulders down. Look straight ahead. Figure 18a.

Slowly turn your head towards your left shoulder as far as is comfortable. Hold for five seconds and return to the starting position. Figure 18b.

Repeat on the right. Figure 18c.

Do three rotations on each side.

Neck stretch

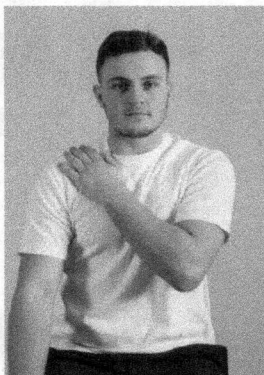

Fig. 19a

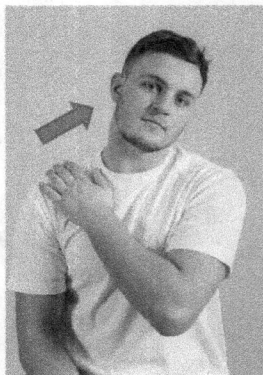

Fig 19b

This stretch is good for loosening tight neck muscles and improving flexibility.
Sitting upright, look straight ahead and hold your right shoulder down with your left hand. Figure 19a.
Slowly tilt your head to the left while holding your shoulder down. Figure 19b.
Repeat on the opposite side.
Hold each stretch for five seconds and repeat three times on each side.

Flexibility Exercises

Sideways bend

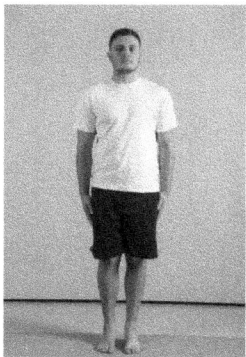 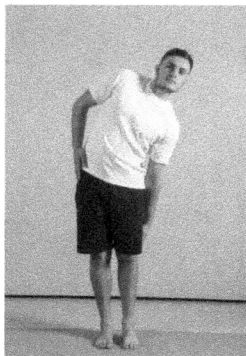 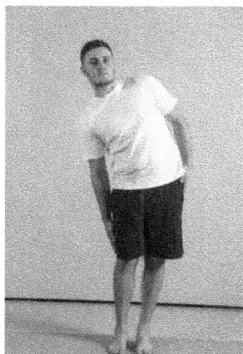

Fig. 20a   Fig. 20b   Fig. 20c

This stretch will help restore flexibility to the lower back.
Stand upright with your arms by your side. Figure 20a.
Slide your left arm down your side as far as is comfortable.
As you lower your arm, you should feel a stretch on the
opposite hip. Figure 20b.
Repeat with your right arm. Figure 20c.
Hold each stretch for five seconds and perform three on each
side.

Calf stretch

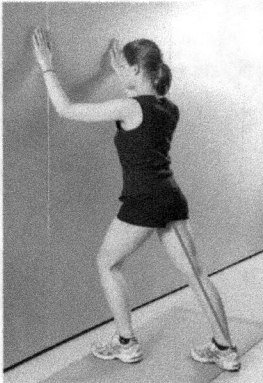
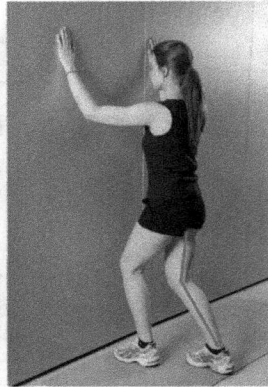

Fig. 21a   Fig 21b

This stretch is good for loosening tight calf muscles.
Place your hands against a wall for stability. Bend the left leg
and step the right leg back at least the length of your foot,
keeping your feet straight. Both feet should be flat on the floor.
The right calf muscle is stretched by keeping the right leg as
straight as possible and the left heel on the floor. Slowly move
your abdomen towards the wall. Figure 21a.
Repeat with the opposite leg. Perform three on each side.
Then, repeat the exercise with the stretched leg in a **bent**
position as illustrated in Figure 21b.

Step-up

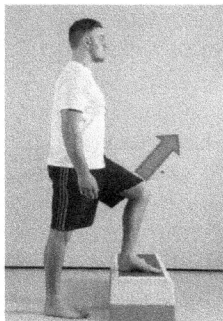
Fig. 22a

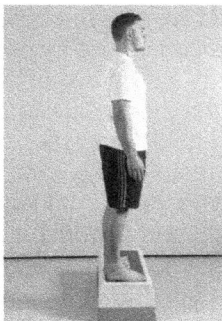
Fig. 22b

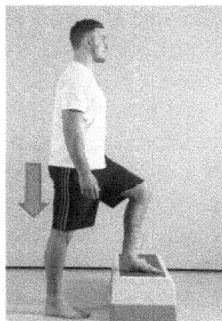
Fig. 22c

Use a step, preferably with a railing or near a wall to use as support.

Step up with your left leg. Figure 22a.

Bring your right leg up to join it. Figure 22b.

Step down again and return to the start position. Figure 22c. The key for building balance is to step up and down **slowly** and in a controlled manner. Perform up to five steps with each leg.

Other Exercises

Toe Taps - Keep your heels on the ground and flex your toes up towards the ceiling and back to the ground. To increase the range of motion, sit towards the edge of a chair with the legs straight and the heel touching the ground. In this position, point the toes down towards the ground and then up towards the ceiling. Repeat these exercises 8 to 10 times. This exercise strengthens the muscles in the lower front and rear of your legs, which you will use for numerous daily activities such as going up and down stairs.

Seated Barbell Twists - A seated barbell twist works your entire core and is an effective chair exercise, provided you move slowly and use a light barbell or similar safe weight (A broom handle will do the trick). Sit with your feet on the floor, your back straight and holding a light barbell across your shoulders. Twist your torso over to your right, pause for five seconds, and then twist over to your left. Figures 23a, b, c. Keep your back straight and abdominals tight throughout the movement. If you do not have a broom handle to hand, simply put your hands behind your head. Figures 23d, e.

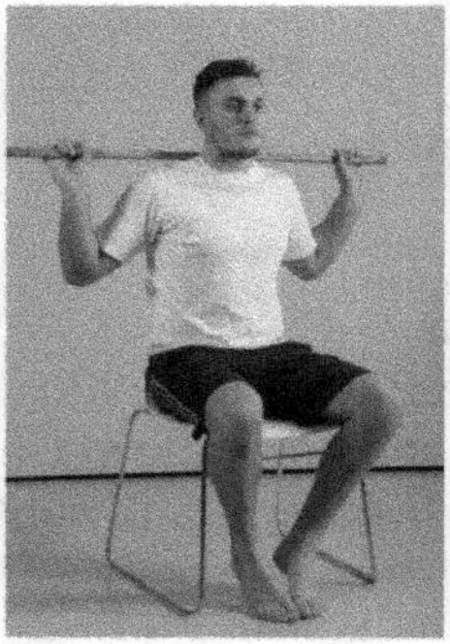

Fig. 23a 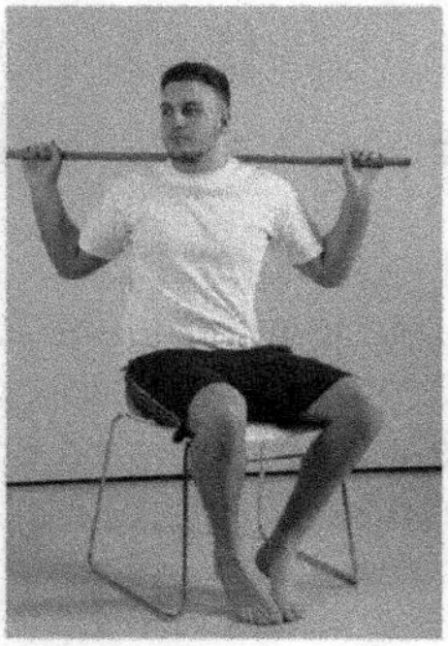   Fig 23b 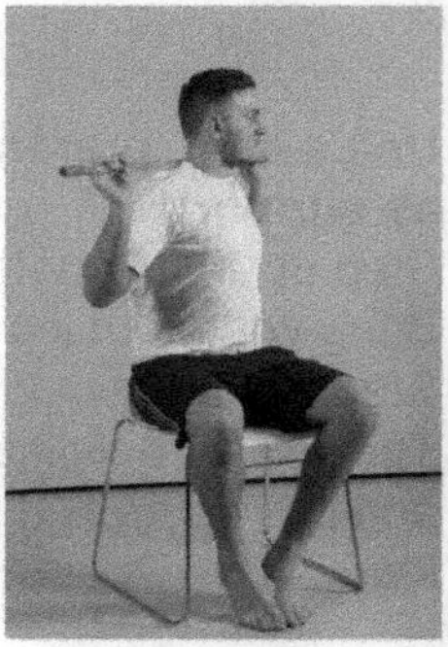   Fig 23c

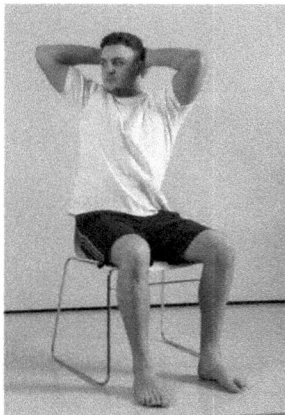 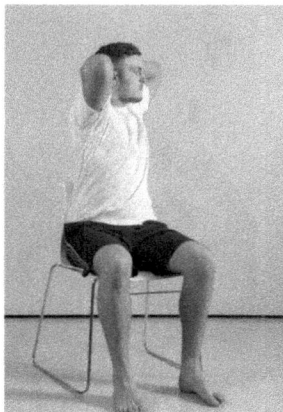

Fig. 23d   *Fig. 23e*

The Vacuum

The vacuum is an isometric abdominal contraction which can help with core muscle development and breathing control. You can perform this exercise standing, lying or seated in a chair. To carry out the exercise, exhale every last bit of air from your lungs. With your chest up and out, suck your stomach in like a vacuum and hold it for 5 to 10 seconds. Figure 24. To give you an idea of how to do the exercise, you could imagine your naval touching your spine.

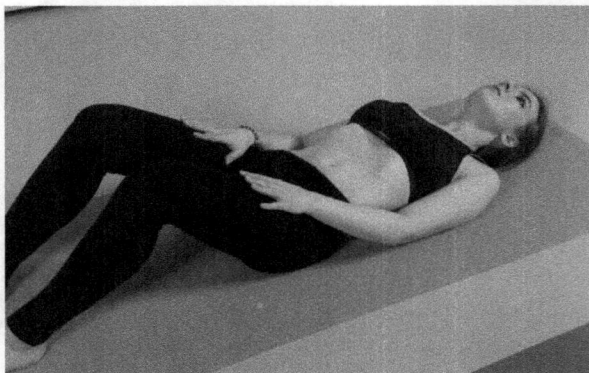

Fig. 24 Vacuum Exercise

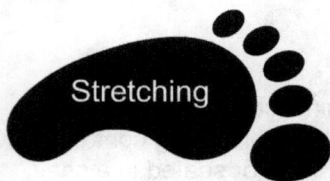

Stretching

The Benefits of Stretching
Stretching results in a number of benefits, such as:

Improving flexibility and energy – Insofar as it improves your physical performance and reduces risk of injury. Flexible muscles are more resistant to injury and damage than inflexible ones. Stretching promotes energy enzymes that can give you a boost during stretching.

Burning calories – An active stretching programme actually burns calories, so you are getting healthier even before you start running.

Reducing the effects of ageing – Stretching can combat inflexibility which is a natural process of ageing. Stretching can improve your range of joint motion, resulting in improved balance, which is important for older people. Improving balance can reduce the potential for falling which is, of course, a big concern in the elderly.

Increasing cardiovascular endurance – Stretching promotes the essential fuelling and oxygenation of the body, helping you prepare for your exercise regime.

Improving the co-ordination of muscle groups – When muscles are regularly, and properly, stretched they adopt a 'second nature' stance. Muscles get used to being extended and contracted in a controlled way and the pathways between your nerves and brain improve. As a result, your body becomes more co-ordinated and your posture and well-being improve.

Alleviating stress – You are able to relax more during a stretch and, moreover, during stretching you forget about your worries as the routines form a 'distraction' from the problems of everyday life.

Improving back pain – Especially, if you stretch in the pelvic and lower back areas, you can 'untangle' the stuck muscles and tendons which, otherwise prevent range of motion.

Elongating muscles – Means you are much less likely to develop injuries. Muscles which are lengthened are more forgiving, allowing you to push your training regime to a higher level.

The emotional angle – Stretching makes you feel better and does your body a power of good.

Warming up

To get the most from your stretching session, it is advisable to warm up properly. You could try some of the gentle flexibility exercises shown earlier in this chapter. Warming up is important as your body functions better when your internal temperature is elevated. Take extra time warming up in cool weather, or when you feel stiff, to reduce the risk of muscle injury.

Which stretches should I do?

There is a plethora of stretching exercise that you could do but, we recommend that you follow these simple stretching exercises, shown in Figure 25, to start with. Please note: It is advisable to perform these stretches gently, without bouncing. It is useful to repeat each stretch about five times and hold (in the stretched position) for 10 seconds.

Stretching

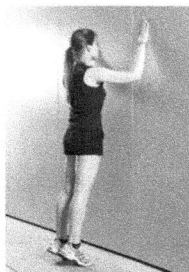

Pectoralis

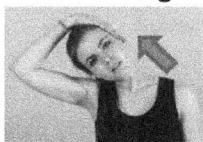

Upper Trapezius

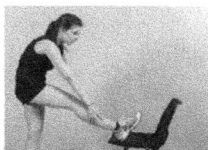

Standing Hamstring

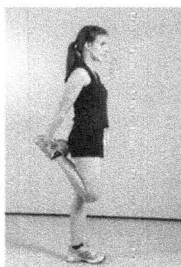

Quadriceps

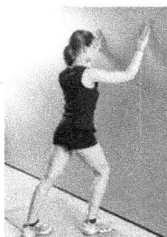

Standing Calf
(Straight)

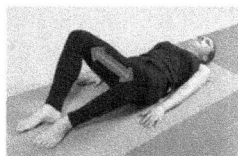

Hip Adductor

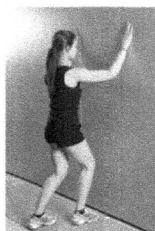

Standing Calf
(Bent)

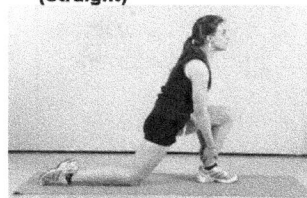

Hip Flexor

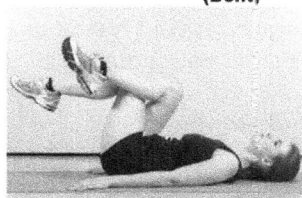

Piriformis

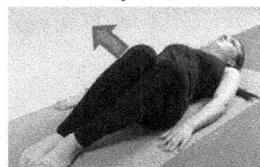

Trunk Rotation

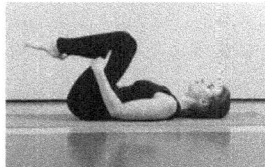

Double Knee to Chest

Fig. 25 Simple Stretching Exercises

77

How to do the stretches shown in Figure 25

Pectoralis
This exercise stretches the pectoralis muscles in the chest and it will help you stand up straighter. Stand facing a wall, with your feet about two foot away from the wall. Place your forearms on the wall at whatever height you find comfortable. Lean in towards the wall until you feel a gentle pull in the front of your chest. You may even feel it in the back of your shoulders or across your shoulder blades.

Upper Trapezius
Keeping your body upright and facing forwards, place the palm of your right hand on the left side of your head and gently pull your head to the right hand side. Repeat on the left.

Standing Hamstring
Stand upright and place your right heel on a stable chair and gently lower your hands down your right leg. You will feel tension in your right leg as your hamstring is stretched.

Quadriceps
Stand on one foot, with one hand on a wall for balance. Hold the other foot with the other hand and raise the heel of the lifted foot to the buttocks (or as close as comfortably possible), stretching your quadriceps. Keep your body upright throughout. Change legs and repeat.

Standing Calf Straight leg
Place your hands against a wall for stability. Bend the right leg and step the left leg back at least the length of your foot, keeping your feet straight. Both feet should be flat on the floor.

The left calf muscle is stretched by keeping the left leg as straight as possible and the right heel on the floor. Slowly move your abdomen towards the wall. Repeat with the opposite leg.

Standing Calf Bent leg
This exercise is similar to the Standing Calf Straight leg, but with the stretched leg in a **bent** position.

Hip Adductor
Lay on your back with your legs together and bring your heels up so that your knees are bent at around 90 degrees. Then start the exercise by gently moving your legs outward so you feel the tension in your groin area. This exercise strengthens your hip adductor muscles.

Hip Flexor
Kneel on your right leg but keep body upright. Hold you left knee with both hands and let your hands slide down your left leg whilst you move your body forwards. You will feel tension in your right hip area.

Piriformis
Lay on the floor on your back and cross the right ankle over the left knee. Grip the thigh of your left leg and pull the knee towards you. Pull the knee further towards you to increase the stretch. This will place tension in your right Pirimormis muscle.

Trunk Rotation
Lay on your back with your legs together and bring your heels up so that your knees are bent at around 90 degrees. Then start the exercise by keeping your knees together and gently moving your legs to the left and then to the right. This

exercise strengthens, and gives mobility to your lower back and hips.

Double Knee to Chest
Lie on your back with your knees bent. Hug your shins to your chest to stretch your hamstrings and lower back.

How often should you stretch?
Ideally, you should stretch every day, but we recognise that this is not always practical. However, please try to stretch as often as your lifestyle allows. This means, taking the opportunity to stretch at your desk, at the bus stop or on your sofa.

When not to stretch
It is best not to stretch when you feel overtired (as you will not be in good alignment) or when you have an injury.

Strength training is an important part of your training and it is sometimes overlooked - It can help with endurance, preventing injury, improving running form and improves bone strength and joint flexibility. And it's not just about strengthening your legs; it includes the whole body such as: arms, core, hips and feet.

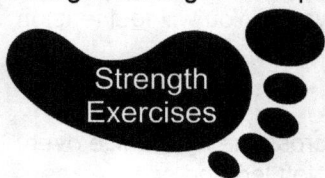

Strength Exercises

There are lots of strength training exercises and various forms of each one you can do, depending on your own strength and ability. You may want to add weights or resistance bands to your strength training.

The first thing to decide is how much time you have for

strength training and whether you will be doing this at home or in the gym. Below are some strength training exercises that you can do in your own home, with no special equipment required, or at your local gym.

Knee Raises - Sit tall in your chair and lift one bent leg at a time toward your chest. At the same time, curl your upper body down to meet your knee. Hold each contraction for five seconds then release and repeat with the other leg. See Figure 26.

Fig. 26 Knee Raises

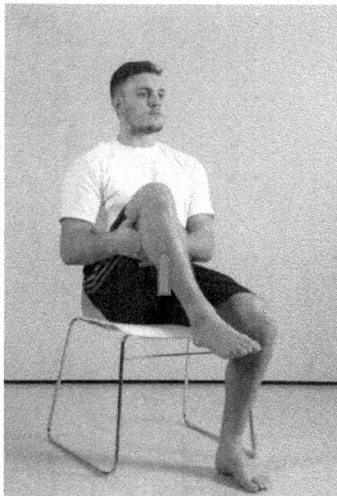

Eccentric Calf Raises - Stretches and strengthens the Achilles tendon, and the two main calf muscles, **gastrocnemius** and **soleus.**

Stand on the stairs with the balls of the foot on the edge (use banisters and walls to steady yourself), then keep both feet level. Lift off one leg and lower the other foot down, stretching out the calf and Achilles (As your full body weight is over your lower limbs, do not over stretch). Hold at the lowest point for 2 seconds then put down the other foot and raise up again onto the balls of both feet. Repeat 5-10 times and then change legs. See Figure 27.

This is great strength training for runners and can, to some extent, prevent Achilles injuries. If this feels too hard then keep both feet on the stair throughout until you get stronger.

As you become more used to doing this exercise you can

alternate the repetitions with a straight leg and a bent leg as you come down. A bent leg will engage the soleus more, while the straight leg will work on the gastrocnemius (the two main muscles in the calf).

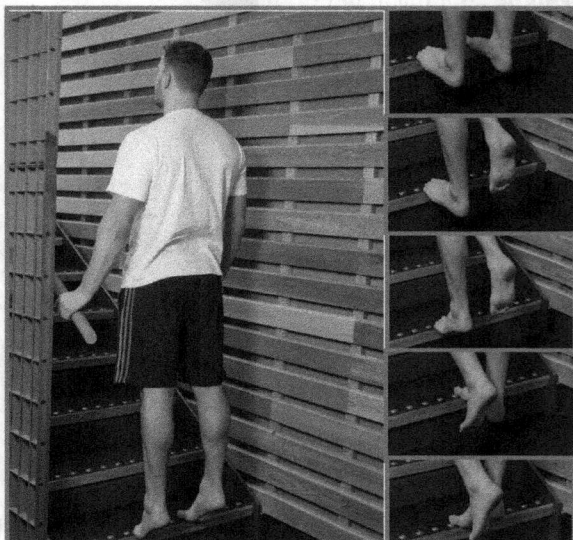

Fig. 27 Eccentric Calf Raises

The Lunge - Good strength training for the knee, as well as quadriceps, hamstrings and lower back.

Stand with your feet shoulder width apart, keeping your back straight. Then with your left leg take a step forward about 3 feet (1 metre), go on to your tip-toes with your right foot and bend your knees to lower your body to the floor, keeping the right knee behind your toes. Straighten your left leg and move back into the starting position. Figure 28.

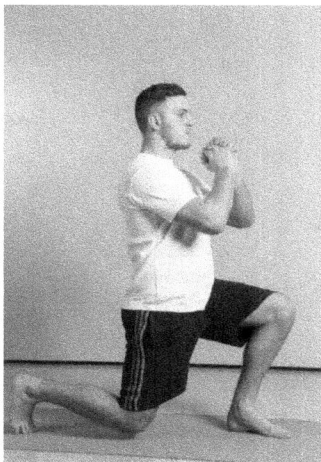

Fig. 28 The Lunge

One Leg Squat - Engages your core muscles, strengthens the quadriceps and gluteus muscles – a great way to build your legs!

Stand on one leg and straighten the other out in front of you. Lift this leg as high as you can without falling backwards, hold your arms to the side for balance if required. Now SLOWLY squat down as far as you can on one leg. Repeat five times then change legs. See Figure 29.

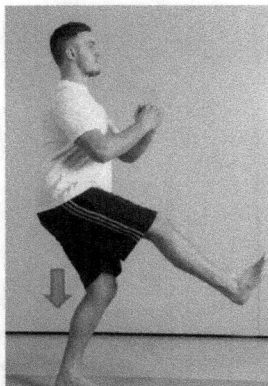

Fig. 29

Side Plank - This is good a core exercise and also strengthens the hips, which is good for your running technique.

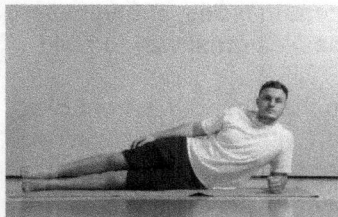

Fig. 30a

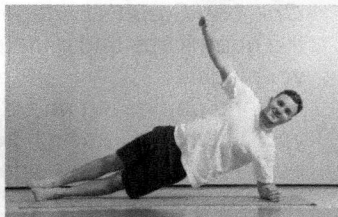

Fig 30b

Lie on left side, resting upper body on left forearm, stretch out legs in a straight line. Figure 30a. Raise up your hips till your body is in a straight line and hold for five seconds. Figure 30b. Then slowly lower back to the start position. Repeat five times then change sides.

Press-Ups - This is good for pectorals, arms and shoulders. If you have never done press ups before, start with your knees on the floor.

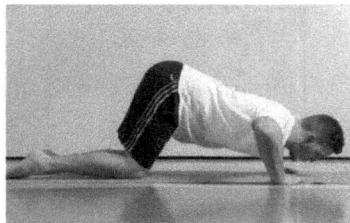 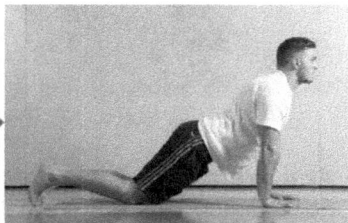

Fig. 31a   *Fig 31b*

With your knees in this position and your nose touching the mat, put your hands in a natural (comfortable) position with your arms bent as shown. Figure 31a. Raise your upper body by straightening your arms and hold for 10 seconds. Figure 31b. Then lower slowly back to the start position. Complete around five of these and gradually increase the number as you get fitter.

As you become stronger, and more confident with this exercise, you can raise your body from your toes, instead of your knees. Figures 32a, b.

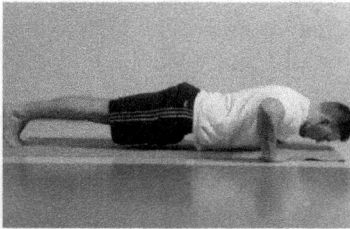
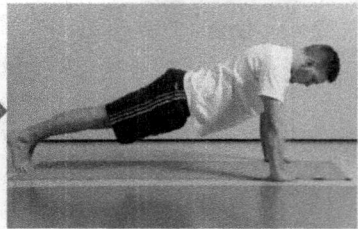

Fig. 32a   *Fig. 32b*

Arm exercises - There are also ways to exercise your arms. For example, there is a small machine known as an *arm cycle* (Ergometer) which can be used while sitting and can help you reap the cardiovascular benefits. There are machines of various grades out there, so it is important to read the reviews. Some are cheaply made pedal machines, while others are made to give very intense aerobic workouts for people who are undergoing rehabilitation. Figure 33 shows and Arm Ergometer in use. It's a great way to get aerobic exercise without having to stand and many gyms have these machines.

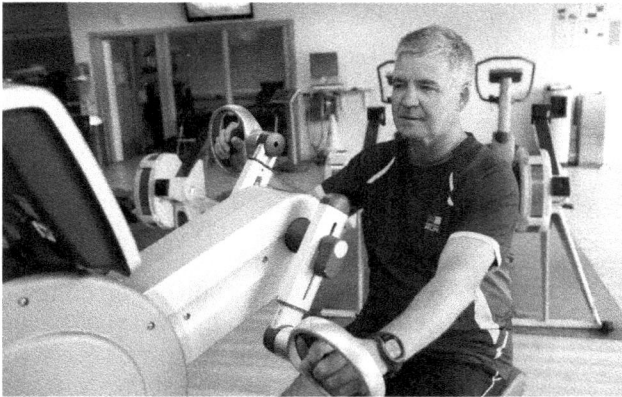

Fig. 33 Arm Ergometer

Your living room is your Gym

You can carry out your exercises easily, without always paying for gym membership, by turning your living room into a mini-gym. You don't need all that expensive equipment normally associated with gyms as you can increase your strength and suppleness at home.

*P*lease be aware of the dangers of using home-made/non-authorised equipment.

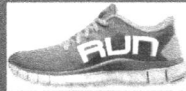

Fitness Training

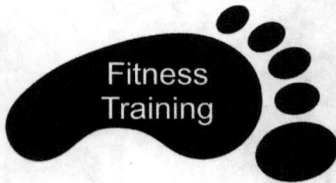

Everyone is totally unique and many runners develop their own style. Take a look at Paula Radcliffe; the World Marathon record holder, despite running with a bobbing head and Alberto Juantorena who seemed to run bow-legged, both beat the competition out of sight. Does style matter and can it/should it be corrected? There are many schools of thought on this, but, we believe that there are some basic style components that might make your running more economical. These are shown in Figure 34 and include:

Head Position - How you hold your head could be important to your overall posture, and may determine how efficiently you run. Try to look ahead naturally, and not down at your feet. This will straighten your neck and back, and bring them more into alignment.

Shoulders - Shoulders play an important role in keeping your upper body relaxed whilst you run, and helps to maintain an efficient running posture. Your shoulders should be low and loose, not high and tight. As you become more tired during a run, try not to let your shoulders creep up towards your ears. If they do, shake them out to release the tension. Your shoulders also need to remain level and shouldn't roll from side to side.

Arms - Arms and hands are important elements in the running process. Your hands control the tension in your upper body, whilst your arm swing works in conjunction with your leg stride to drive you forward. It is good to keep your hands in an unclenched fist, with your fingers lightly touching your palms. Your arms should swing mostly forward and back, not across your body, between waist and lower-chest level. Your elbows should be bent at about a 90-degree angle. When you feel your fists clenching or your forearms tensing up, try to drop your arms down to your sides and shake them out for a few seconds to release the tension.

Torso - Try to run upright to promote efficient breathing and to lengthen your stride. This position is described as 'running tall' and it means you are stretching yourself up to your full height with your back comfortably straight. If, during a run, you start to slouch take a deep breath and feel yourself naturally straighten again.

Hips - Your hips are said to be your centre of gravity. With your torso and back comfortably upright and straight, your hips should naturally fall into proper alignment, to point you in a straight ahead position. If you allow your torso to hunch over or lean too far forward during a run, your pelvis will tilt forward as well, which can put pressure on your lower back and throw the rest of your lower body out of alignment.

Legs/Stride - Sprinters generally need to lift their knees high to achieve maximum leg power, whereas distance runners don't need such an exaggerated knee lift as it becomes too hard to sustain for any length of time. Efficient endurance running requires just a slight knee lift, a quick leg turnover, and a short stride. As your foot strikes the ground, your knee should be slightly flexed so that it can bend naturally on impact.

Ankles/Feet - To run well, you need to push off the ground with maximum force. With each stride, your foot should hit the ground lightly, landing between your heel and mid-foot, then quickly rolling forward to your toes. If you strike heel first then you are, in effect, putting the brakes on. It is advisable to keep your ankle flexed as your foot rolls forward to create more force for push-off. As you roll onto your toes, try to spring off the ground. Try not to slap loudly as your feet hit the ground as good running should be springy and quiet.

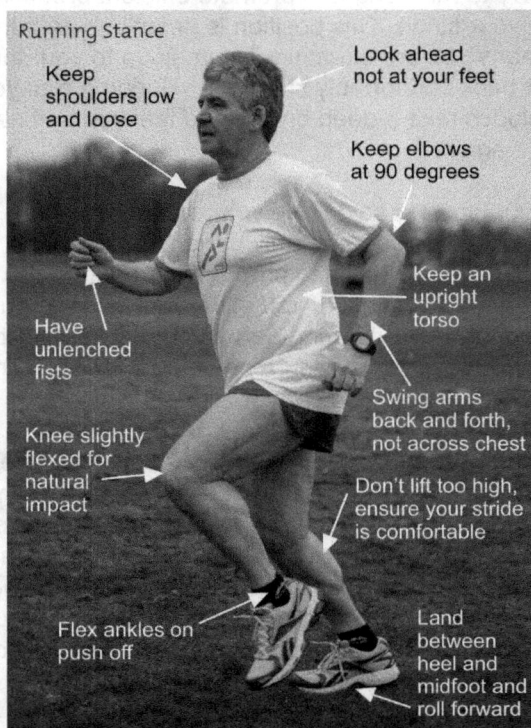

Running Stance

Keep shoulders low and loose

Look ahead not at your feet

Keep elbows at 90 degrees

Keep an upright torso

Have unlenched fists

Swing arms back and forth, not across chest

Knee slightly flexed for natural impact

Don't lift too high, ensure your stride is comfortable

Flex ankles on push off

Land between heel and midfoot and roll forward

Fig. 34 Running Stance

The psychological connection
There is such a close link between our mind and our body that, if you feel tired you may run uneconomically, you may be in a slouched position and, as a result, may feel de-motivated. However, if you raise your head and look up, you might have a different perspective, will feel better and start to run more economically.

Energy Systems occurring during fitness training
Whilst this book is not a science text, we wanted to provide some information about how energy works on our bodies.

A runner's body is capable of using one or a combination of three energy systems. Different running disciplines (e.g. sprinting, 5k running, marathons) demand different types and amounts of muscle activity. Therefore, different energy systems are predominant in the various disciplines. Improving running performance, therefore, can be achieved by carefully designed training schedules that increase the utilisation of specific energy systems and muscle groups as shown in Figure 35.

In essence, if oxygen (or air), is required for running then the energy system is **aerobic**. If oxygen is not required, the system is **anaerobic**. In addition, if lactic acid is produced, then the system is **lactic**. If not, and no air is required, it is an **alactic** system. Marathon runners, for example, produce most of their energy aerobically, while sprinters and field event athletes depend more on anaerobic sources. This aerobic/anaerobic ratio is determined by identifying how long and how hard runners work without rest.

Consider Figure 35, from left to right there is an **Alactic System (anaerobic)**. This is the stored, start-up system which does not require oxygen and does not produce lactic acid. Then, there is the **Anaerobic Lactic (or Lactate) System**. In this, the system does not require oxygen but produces lactic acid. And finally, there is an **Aerobic System**, or the muscle energy system, which requires oxygen.

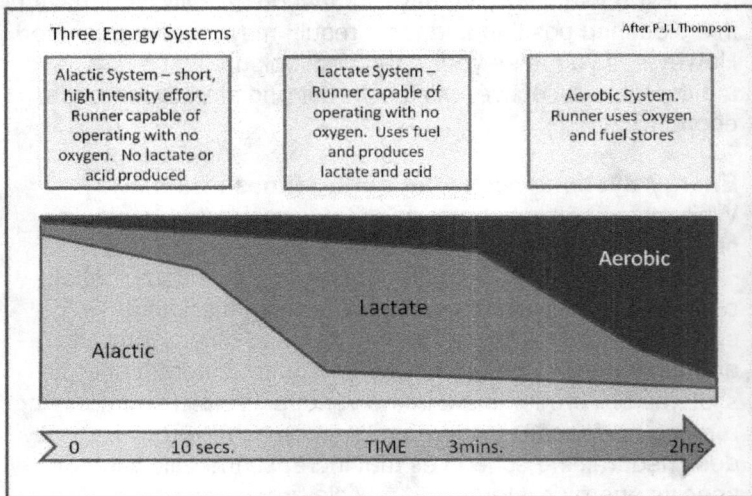

Three Energy Systems — After P.J.L Thompson

Alactic System – short, high intensity effort. Runner capable of operating with no oxygen. No lactate or acid produced

Lactate System – Runner capable of operating with no oxygen. Uses fuel and produces lactate and acid

Aerobic System. Runner uses oxygen and fuel stores

Aerobic

Lactate

Alactic

0   10 secs.   TIME   3mins.   2hrs.

Fig. 35 Three Energy Systems

Alactic (anaerobic) Energy System

The anaerobic alactic system is the one referred to as the stored or start up energy system. This system provides most of the energy when runners do bursts of high speed or high resistance movements lasting up to 10 seconds. The stores of energy in the muscle which are used up in the intense burst of activity return to normal levels within 2-3 minutes of rest.

Lactate (Anaerobic) Energy System

This energy system is capable of high levels of intensity, but this intensity prevents the removal of waste products as insufficient oxygen is available. As a result, lactic acid accumulates within muscle cells and blood. This is a major cause of fatigue, eventually slowing the runner down. The more intense the exercise rate, the faster the rate of lactic acid accumulation, leading to fatigue. For example, a 400 metre sprinter will accumulate high levels of lactic acid after 35-40 seconds. Whereas, an 800 metre runner, going slightly slower, accumulates lactic acid at a slower rate, reaching high levels after about 70-85 seconds. Eliminating lactic acid after running is a much slower process than the replacement of energy stores in the anaerobic alactic system.

Aerobic System

The aerobic system requires oxygen. This system is used in lower intensity exercise and is the basic system which provides the energy for most human activity. It is a very efficient system and does not produce fatigue-producing waste products. The heart and lungs are important in aerobic activity as oxygen and fuel need to be transported, in the blood, to the muscles. The aerobic system resists fatigue and takes longer to overload than the anaerobic systems. Training the aerobic energy system would normally be a minimum of 20 minutes duration and, the work load for aerobic training can be either continuous or broken into intervals.

Training to a schedule

Many runners train to a schedule and embrace a monthly, weekly or even daily pattern. This is often the case when runners are training for a specific event like a sprint, a 10k or a marathon. A schedule can be helpful because it imparts a certain discipline for the runner and can help them to focus on specific goals.

Whatever your level of fitness you should comfortably be able to build from nothing to running continuously for 30 minutes in the space of around eight weeks. All you need to do is make a commitment to run at least three times a week and follow this simple run-walk programme which will gradually ease you towards your fitness goal (as outlined in Chapter 4).

The basic Schedule:

- **Week 1** Run 1 minute, walk 90 seconds. Repeat 8 times, 3 times a week.
- **Week 2** Run 2 mins, walk 1 min. Repeat 7 times, 3 times a week.
- **Week 3** Run 3 mins, walk 1 min. Repeat 6 times, 3 times a week.
- **Week 4** Run 5 mins, walk 2 mins. Repeat 4 times, 3 times a week.
- **Week 5** Run 8 mins, walk 2 mins. Repeat 3 times, 3 times a week.
- **Week 6** Run 12 mins, walk 1 min. Repeat 3 times, 3 times a week.
- **Week 7** Run 15 mins, walk 1 min, Repeat 3 times, 3 times a week
- **Week 8** Run 30 minutes continuously. Good luck!

As you become fitter, more advanced training schedules can be found at:
http://www.runnersworld.co.uk/racing/find-a-training-plan/4521.html or, you can create your own schedule to suit your current needs and future goals.

A few things you might want to bear in mind:

- Respecting your body and how you feel is the best route

to fitness. Getting fit should NOT be a punishment.

- When you begin to train to a schedule, it is good to allow at least one day's rest between runs.
- If you feel tired then just slow down a bit. Ideally, you should be able to hold a conversation whilst running.
- When you walk, do it purposefully and be strict with your run/walk timings.
- Don't be afraid to repeat one of the weekly schedules, or, even revert back to one of the previous week's activities.

Awareness of your Heart/Pulse rate

Some runners prefer to run to a pre-determined Heart/Pulse rate and that is why Heart Rate Monitors are so popular.

Training to a heart rate can help you to maximise your fitness. It is generally agreed that 220 beats per minute (bpm) minus your age is a good guide to fitness. For example if you are 40 years of age, your ideal training heart/pulse rate would be 220-40 = 180bpm.

This is a general rule, however, and if you would like to have a more specific heart rate measurement then, we recommend that you see a fitness Instructor, at your local gym, for a treadmill test. This test typically involves you running on a treadmill whilst being connected to a monitor to record your heart rate. The test may also record your blood pressure and your Oxygen consumption. Even with an accurate heart rate reading, there still may be limitations when you're using a heart rate monitor to determine your work rate.

Typical heart rate monitors (HRM) are easy to fit, are quite comfortable to wear and can give you instant feedback on your progress during a training run. It is not essential to use a HRM but, if you are interested and would find it useful to keep an eye on your pulse, you could just take a reading during, or at the end of your exercise session.

Cool Down

The idea of a Cool Down is to allow your whole body to return to a relaxed state after exertion. It is advisable after a training run or race to do some stretching exercises. This is to loosen the body and help prevent tightness occurring in the muscles. Exercises, such as those illustrated earlier, should help to reduce tightness. Once again, it is important to ease into any stretching routine (do not over stretch).

Following a race and before you get into your car, go to the presentation, or have a well-earned drink; put on another layer of clothing (adjust according to the weather conditions) and just relax. Although you may not feel like doing a 'Cool Down' after a race or a training run, its benefits are well worth the effort.

The Treadmill alternative

Why use a Treadmill? - If the weather outside is really icy, snowy or rainy, or if you just fancy an indoor run, you could use a treadmill. Treadmills provide a useful complement to your running and fitness programme. They are useful if you are recovering from injury and just want to test out your rehabilitation stage (You can stop at any point, without being stranded miles from home). They are a good means of checking out your form, or alignment, in front of a mirror and they are invaluable if you live near busy roads and just want to feel safer. Martin and Geoff often use treadmills if they are away on business, or at a holiday location with no suitable running terrain.

Treadmills have continuous bands rotating on a platform below your feet. This gives the effect of the ground moving whilst you remain in the same place. Treadmills are readily available at gym clubs or, you may have one in your home. Figure 36 shows a treadmill in use and we advise these simple guidelines to make your treadmill running effective, enjoyable and safe.

Safety first - Please **do not** hold onto the handrails. They are only there to help you get safely on and off the treadmill. Also, many treadmills have auto cut-off devices that stop the machine instantly, if you fall over. Therefore, look for the big red Crocodile clip and attach it to your clothing.

Warm-up - It is very tempting to jump on the treadmill and start your workout at full speed, but you should allow time for a warm up. To warm up you could run or walk at a steady pace for up to 10 minutes and see this as an essential part of your indoor workout.

Set the incline - As there is no wind resistance indoors, you could opt to set the inclination of the treadmill to 1% or 2%. A gentle uphill also simulates outdoor running. However, if this feels too much in the early days of your fitness programme, then leave the treadmill level to begin with. We also recommend that, if you do use an incline, you keep it to less than 6%. Otherwise, this could put excessive strain on your calf or Achilles areas.

Run using good form - Once on the treadmill and, having set the required incline, practice good upper body form, just as you would if running outdoors, by keeping your head up and your arms at 90 degrees. It is not necessary to lean forwards too much because the action of the treadmill naturally pulls your feet backwards. You also need to pull your feet off the belt before they are driven away by the belt's linear action. This may take a bit of getting used to.

Try to look forwards because, but if you are looking down, your running form may be compromised. Try not to stare at your feet as you may be prone to running in a hunched position, which could lead to back and neck pain.

Stride pattern - Keep your stride quick and short in order

to minimise any impact being transferred to your legs. Try to maintain a mid-foot stance to prevent heel-striking sending shock to your knee joints. You may find that you need to exaggerate heel lift, as the lack of forward momentum means your feet will not be moving in a circular motion.

The more steps you take per minute, the more efficiently you'll run. Some experienced runners take about 180 steps per minute and you can determine your stride count by counting how often one foot hits the belt in a given minute and times it by two. Try to improve your stride count during your run by focusing on taking shorter, quicker strides and keeping your feet close to the belt. This technique may even improve your outdoor running.

The concentration factor - Treadmill running should only be conducted for relatively short times (30 minutes is a good maximum guideline) as it can become tedious. To pass the time on a treadmill you could try visualising an outdoor route that you frequently run on. Just picture yourself as you pass well-known landmarks.

Keeping cool and hydrated - Since there is little air resistance to help keep you cool, you may perspire even more running on a treadmill than you would if you were outdoors. Therefore, have a drinks bottle and towel within easy reach.

Cooling off - As you come to the end of your treadmill workout, your heart rate will be elevated. Therefore, don't simply jump off the machine, instead spend five or more minutes doing a slow run or walk, at the end of your session, to allow your heart rate to return below 100 bpm. Cooling down will help prevent you feeling dizzy and will reduce the feeling that you're still moving when you step off the treadmill. As a courtesy to other gym users it is good practice to wipe down the machine after use.

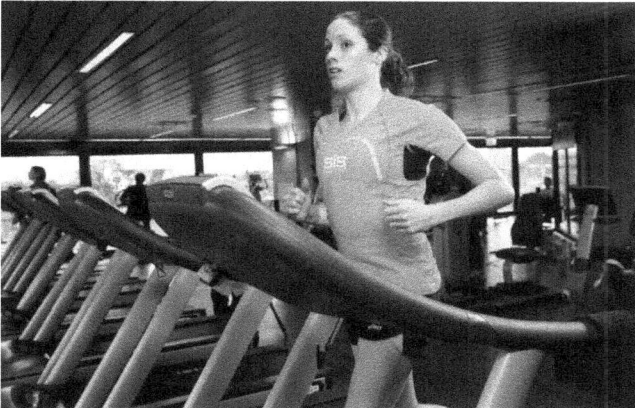

Fig. 36 Treadmill Training. Image provided by SiS and reproduced by kind permission of Helen Jenkins (World Triathlon Champion).

High Intensity Training (HIT)

Why?

If you are' time-poor', for example if you travel a lot for your job or you have many demanding commitments, it is st ll possible to gain some benefits from exercise by using a High Intensity Training (HIT) regime. HIT is a time-efficient alternative to traditional exercise but it is also very fatiguing. However, some of the proven benefits of High Intensity Training include:

- Time savings
- Improved aerobic fitness and endurance
- Reduced body fat
- Increased upper and lower body strength

What is HIT?

High Intensity Training was around in the 1970s and was aimed primarily at body builders. However, since 2011 HIT has become more popular as a cardiovascular exercise for athletes, but the principles remain similar and simple: HIT consists of a few relatively short bursts of intense exercise, adding up to only a few minutes commitment each week.

HIT is relatively simple and can be carried out by running (on the spot), running up stairs or cycling on a static machine. For example, you can get on an exercise bike and warm up for a few minutes by doing some gentle cycling, then cycle at very high speed for twenty seconds. After that take two minutes to recover and get your breath back before cycling for another 20 seconds at very high intensity. Finally, have another two minutes of very gentle cycling, then a final 20-second burst, going as fast as possible. Have a two minute gentle cool down session and your total exercise time is around 10 minutes.

How does it work?

HIT gets your heart rate up, maintains the rate and burns more fat in less time. This kind of workout increases your body's need for oxygen during the effort and creates an oxygen shortage, causing your body to require more oxygen during recovery. This effect may help to burn more fat and calories than regular aerobic and steady-state workouts. HIT also utilises more of our muscle tissue than classic aerobic exercise. When you perform a HIT workout, you are not just using your leg muscles, but also your upper body, arms and shoulders. In this way around 80% of the body's muscle cells are activated, compared to 20-40% for walking or moderate intensity jogging or cycling. *Ref: Jamie Timmons, professor of ageing biology, Birmingham University.* Active exercise, like

HIT, can also break down the body's stores of glucose, stored as glycogen in our muscles and helps in the overall fitness cycle.

Are there any risks?
As with any form of high-intensity activity, it is useful to have a health check before embarking on HIT. Furthermore, HIT puts a lot of stress on your cardiovascular system so you need to be in reasonable shape to conduct this type of activity. Make sure you stretch properly and start slowly to reduce the risk of injury. HIT has its place in the wider repertoire of training schedules and could be beneficial for people without much spare time. HIT works better when combined with other training programmes, but it might not bring the other wider benefits of fitness and exercise as outlined in chapters 1 to 3.

What about the science?
As we mentioned earlier in this book, we do not want to be overly scientific but, for interest, Richard S. Metcalfe *etal* published a paper in July 2012 in The European Journal of Applied Physiology, relating to the effects of high-intensity interval training.

Running Injuries
Running Injuries do occur from time to time and, actually, are not untypical of the fitness process. Therefore, if you do get injured, it is important to remember that a vital part of recovery is in **accepting the injury**. The most common running injuries are shown in figure 37.

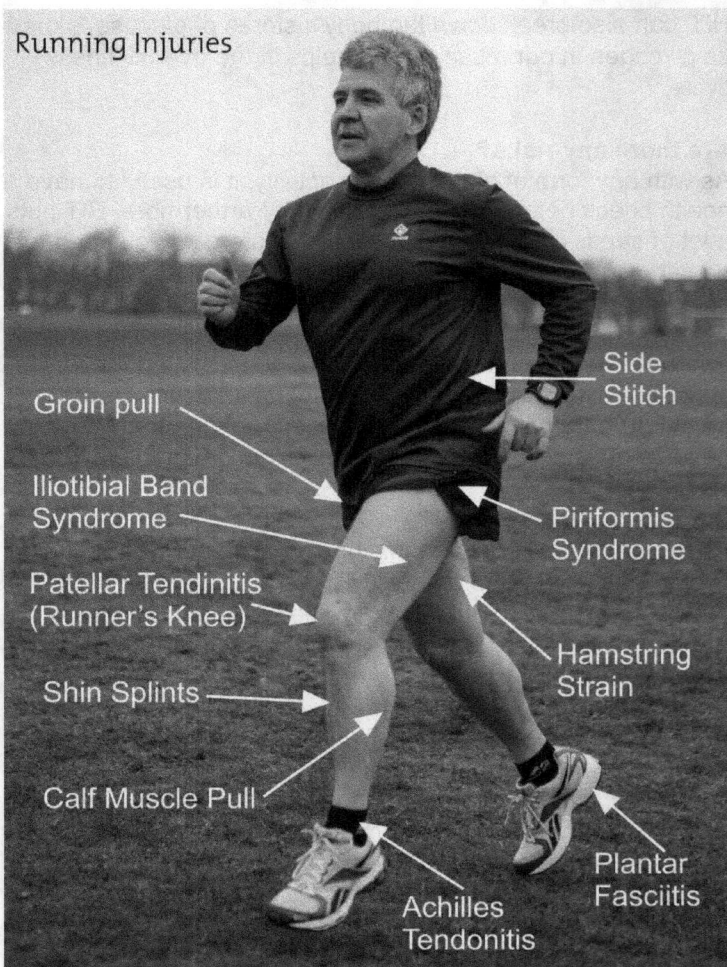

Fig. 37 Common Running Injuries

Injuries explained

- **Runner's knee** is where you experience a tender pain around or behind the patella (or kneecap) and is a sure sign of patellofemoral pain, otherwise known as Runners Knee. The repetitive force of pounding on the pavement, downhill running, muscle imbalances, and weak hips can put extra stress on the patella, so try softer running surfaces and flat ground wherever possible. To treat the pain you could try knee taping, anti-inflammatory medications, specific stretches and reducing your mileage.

- **Achilles tendinitis** is the swelling of the Achilles, the tissues that connect the heel to lower-leg muscles, and can be the result of many factors: rapid mileage increase, improper footwear or tight calf muscles. Make sure to always stretch the calf muscles after a workout, and wear supportive shoes. Also, reduce the hill climbing, which puts extra stress on tendons. Anti-inflammatories, stretching, or R.I.C.E strategy (see further in this chapter), are the best ways to get back on the path to recovery.

- **Plantar fasciitis** is due to the inflammation, irritation, or tearing of the plantar fascia-tissue on the bottom of the foot. The main cause is excess pounding on the roads, extreme stiffness or a stabbing pain in the arch of the foot. Wearing shoes with extra cushioning, stretching, rolling a tennis ball or golf ball over the heel, and getting plenty of rest can help dull the pain.

- **Iliotibial band syndrome** triggers pain on the outside of the knee, due to inflammation of the Iliotibial band, a thick tendon that stretches from the pelvic bone down the tibia. Common causes include increased mileage, downhill running or weak hips. To ease the pain, do some specific stretches, along with foam rolling (rollers available from sports outlets) as this can decrease inflammation and help reduce pain.

- **Stress fractures** are tiny cracks in the bone caused by repeatedly pounding greater amounts of force than the leg bones can bear. Taking some time off is a must and you may need to use some supports alongside physical therapy. In some cases, an x-ray may be required to fully assess any damage. To avoid being side-lined, build in plenty of cross-training to avoid overuse injuries, wear good shoes and ensure you are getting sufficient calcium to keep your bones strong.

- **Patellar tendinitis** is common amongst distance runners and strikes when overuse leads to tiny tears in the patellar tendon (the tendon that connects the kneecap to the shinbone). Overpronation, over-training, and too many hill repeats are likely causes. To reduce the risk of patellar tendinitis, it is good to strengthen the hamstrings and quadriceps and ice the knee at the onset of pain. You could also have some physical therapy to help soothe and strengthen the tendon.

- **Shin splints** are among the most nagging of injuries, shin splints occur when the muscles and tendons covering the shinbone become inflamed. Try icing the shins for 15-20 minutes and keeping them elevated at night to reduce swelling. Some runners find that shock-absorbing insoles supporting the arch may help. Also stick to running on softer ground whenever possible and avoid hills as these put extra force on the Tibialis muscle.

• **Ankle sprain** is where the ankle rolls in or outward, stretching the ankle ligament (and causing serious pain). Kerbs, potholes and tree branches can be just a few of the unfortunate hazards leading to ankle injuries. Recovery may take a little while at first, but many physiotherapists suggest doing balance exercises to strengthen the muscles around the ankle. Take some rest after the sprain occurs and visit a physiotherapist to agree a recovery plan. They might also recommend an ankle brace or cast and taping it up when you're ready to get back running to prevent reoccurrence.

• **Pulled muscles** are when a muscle is overstretched, fibres and tendons can tear and cause a pulled muscle. Overuse, inflexibility, and not warming-up properly are a few probable causes. A well-considered warm-up, cool-down, and stretching pre-workout is the best way to avoid a muscle pull. Whilst the pain persists, lay off running and stick to gentle stretching and icing of the muscle.

• **Side stitch or Runners Stitch** is that nagging pain on the side of your stomach and was previously called exercise-related transient abdominal pain (ETAP). Side stitches can really creep up on you, affecting nearly 70 per cent of runners. Experts believe the pain is caused by the diaphragm beginning to spasm due to overwork and they also suggest that poor running posture could be to blame. If a stitch strikes, try bending forward and tightening the core, or breathing out to ease the pain.

*M*artin regularly ran the Burnsall 10-mile road race. This is a challenging course in beautiful Dales countryside. He often found himself contracting a stitch in this particular race (we think he was trying too hard) and he had to lean over and exhale a few times during the event to shake off the side pain.

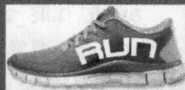

- **Blisters** can appear when we least expect them. Heels rub against the shoe, the top layer of skin can tear and leave a bubble between the layers of skin. The best thing to do is to make sure the shoe fits properly and wear a good pair of socks. There are many anti-blister socks on the market. If a blister still appears, cover it up with blister packs or gels.

- **Chafing** for most, there's no escaping it. When skin rubs against skin, or when clothes rub against skin, the skin can become angry and irritated. You could find clothing that fits well and you can use lubricants to reduce the risk of chafing. Try Vaseline or Glide.

Injury prevention
Prevention is better than cure!

There is no doubt that with a little understanding of how our bodies work we can take steps to reduce the possibility of injuries as we embark on our running journey. Some suppleness and strength training can complement your running on your journey to increased fitness. Please see the flexibility/suppleness exercises and stretches earlier in this chapter.

Also, to prevent injury it is advisable to run on surfaces with not too much camber (avoiding ankle sprains). You should also make sure that you have warmed up before your exercise routine. Regularly check your footwear and replace your training shoes if they are showing excessive signs of wear.

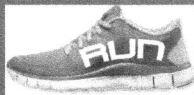

*M*artin and Geoff regularly visit a masseuse to have a leg massage to keep their muscles and soft tissues in tip top condition.

If injuries do occur – don't give up and do not be put off by initial aches and pains. These are normal consequences of re-starting, or commencing, a fitness programme. Minor aches and pains are your body's way of congratulating you for having a go at improving your fitness.

If you do become injured, a valid first intervention might be to apply the **RICE** method. This stands for:

Rest – just take some time out and give your body a chance to heal.

Ice – to promote blood flow, apply an ice pack to the affected area. Please note not to put frozen packs directly next to the skin as this can cause serious burns. It is best to wrap the ice pack in a thin towel.

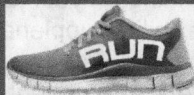

hen icing a sore muscle, Geoff uses a bag of frozen peas. This is an inexpensive means of applying ice and, moreover, the bag will assume the shape of your injured area.

Compression (or comfortable support) – apply a compression bandage/support around the affected area to limit swelling.

Elevation – keep the injured area raised above the level of your heart. This may also help to reduce swelling.

However, if the injury does persist then we suggest that you seek a professional opinion. You could ask the specialists at your local running club or you could check out your symptoms and find a recommended physiotherapist at www.csp.org.uk. If, for some reason you are not satisfied with the service you receive then you could always seek a second opinion. For example, Paula Radcliffe consulted around 10 specialists before she found the root cause of her foot injury. Reference: Paula, My Story So Far ISBN: 0-7434-7869-X. You may wish to try a few specialists until you find the one that suits you.

YOU ARE WHAT YOU EAT ... AND DRINK

Introduction

Now that you are up and running and starting to enjoy the benefits of this amazing sport, we can start to think about how improving nutrition can support your running and deliver you all the benefits that you are looking for. Diet and Nutrition are important because research shows that the prevalence of obesity in many parts of the world has risen significantly over the past few decades.* This has prompted efforts from governments to increase awareness about the importance of a balanced diet and staying physically active in order to maintain a healthy weight and optimum physical and mental health.

Whether you are just trying to get started at incorporating exercise into your lifestyle, or you are a body builder or a professional athlete, **nutrition and hydration play a key role** in physical activity and training, providing you with the fuel you need in order to carry out your exercise.

In this chapter we describe the key components, or nutrients, of foods and explain how they are important for exercise and fitness.

The basics - Energy

Energy is measured in **calories** (The amount of energy, or heat, it takes to increase the temperature of 1 gram of water by 1 degree Celsius), and is how our intake of food is calculated. On average, a man needs around 2,500 calories a day to function well and maintain a healthy weight, and a woman needs around 2,000 calories per day. These amounts are just approximates and can vary depending on a person's age, level of physical activity and other factors.

Often, when individuals are trying to get fit and maintain a healthy weight they can become focused on monitoring their calorie consumption. However, it is important to remember that eating a healthy and balanced diet, staying physically active and balancing the calorie intake with those burned is also important.

Calories and Kilocalories (kcal)
It's easy to get confused about calories and kilocalories since, in a nutritional context, values are actually given for the number of kilocalories in a food, but referred to simply as calories.

In scientific terms:
1000 calories = 1 kilocalorie = 1 kcal.

In nutrition terms ie. What you'll find on food packaging:
Calories = kilocalories and are used interchangeably.

Nutrients
Nutrients are components in foods that an organism uses to survive and grow. Nutrients include; carbohydrates, fats, proteins and vitamins. The calories we do consume must provide a good energy and nutrient balance and, ideally the average day-to-day diet should include the following nutrients:

- Carbohydrates – these are our key energy source.
- Fats – another key energy source important in relation to fat soluble vitamins.
- Proteins – needed for the growth and repair of muscles and body tissue.
- Minerals – inorganic elements which occur in the body.

- Roughage – the fibrous portion of our diet which is needed for a healthy digestive system.
- Vitamins – water soluble and fat soluble vitamins are important in many of the body's chemical processes.
- Water – carries other nutrients around the body and is required for normal body functioning.

Carbohydrates

There are two key forms of carbohydrates – simple sugars and complex (starchy). Simple sugars are carbohydrates which are found in refined sugars and provide a sweet taste. These are naturally found in milk products, fruit and vegetables but can also be added to foods using white sugar, brown sugar, honey, molasses and maple syrup etc.

Though all of the sugars which we eat (whether they occur naturally or are added) are used by the body in the same way, it is better to get your simple sugars from foods in which they occur naturally, as these foods also contain fibre and important nutrients.

Complex carbohydrates, also known as starches, include grains such as bread, pasta and rice. As with simple sugars there are some complex carbohydrates which are better than others, with processed refined grains such as white rice and white flour being less favourable as the nutrients and fibre are removed. Nutritionists recommend that where possible, individuals should consume unrefined grains which are still packed full of vitamins, minerals and fibre.

The carbohydrates we consume are then converted into glucose, a form of sugar which is carried in the blood and delivered to the cells for energy. When this happens the glucose is then broken down into water and carbon dioxide. Any that is unused will be converted into glycogen, another form of carbohydrate that is stowed away in the muscles and liver. The body is unable to hold any more than around 350 grams of glycogen at any one point, and once it has reached full capacity, any excess glucose will be converted into fat.

Glycogen is energy which is stored within the body and used as fuel during exercise, whilst also helping to maintain water. Some long distance athletes will use a technique known as *carbohydrate-loading*. This essentially means they stock up on carbohydrates to increase the amount of glycogen available for a long event, and rely on the slow release of glycogen to fuel the body in the later stages of the race.

Fats

Fat is an essential component of any diet as it helps the body to absorb nutrients. It is also a great source of energy providing the body with essential fatty acids that it is unable to manufacture independently. However, though fats are important we should attempt to monitor how much of them we are eating, as large amounts could lead to excess weight gain and could subsequently result in an increased risk of serious health concerns such as heart disease and high blood pressure.

All fat contains both saturated and unsaturated fatty acids though and are usually referred to as either 'saturated' or 'unsaturated' depending on the percentage of fatty acids present. Saturated fats are commonly found in animal products and processed foods such as meat, dairy and chips, and unsaturated fats are found in foods such as avocados, olives, nuts and oily fish.

Saturated fat is not considered to be healthy for the heart and is known to raise LDL (Low Density Lipoprotein) (bad) cholesterol levels. Unsaturated fats, on the other hand, are considered to be heart healthy and can actually work to lower your LDL cholesterol levels as well as raising your HDL (good) cholesterol levels.

Just to recap, cholesterol is carried in the blood attached to proteins called lipoproteins. There are two main forms, LDL (Low Density Lipoprotein) and HDL (High Density Lipoprotein). LDL cholesterol is often referred to as bad cholesterol because too much is unhealthy. HDL is often referred to as 'good cholesterol' because it is protective as described in Chapter 2.

Protein

Protein is present in every cell of the body and is important for helping to build and repair tissues. It is also used to make enzymes, hormones and a variety of additional body chemicals as well as forming the building blocks of bones, muscles, cartilage, skin and blood. Similar to carbohydrates and fats, protein is a macronutrient and the body requires a large amount of it, but unlike fat and carbohydrates, the body has nowhere to store protein for when it requires a new supply. Therefore it is important to control the intake of protein foods. These include meat, fish, eggs, pulses, nuts, seeds and soya products. The balanced, healthy eating plate is shown in Figure 38.

A balanced plate:

1. Fruit and vegetables
2. Cereals, grains and potatoes
3. Dairy
4. Eggs, fish, meat and nuts
5. Fats and sugars

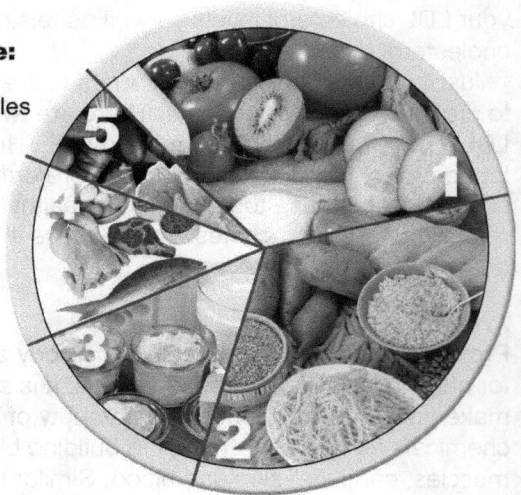

Fig. 38 Balanced Food Plate

Energy Requirements for Exercise

If you are doing a lot of exercise or training regularly your body will need more energy than it would if you were doing nothing. During exercise your heart will beat faster in order to pump blood more rapidly around the body, the lungs work harder and your muscles will contract and expand. All of this will use up your stored energy at a faster rate than normal and you will need to consume the right amount of food each day so that what you eat and what you burn remains in balance.

As you start your training regime you should not use this as a licence to gorge on unhealthy foods, but aim to optimise portion sizes of carbohydrate-rich foods such as porridge, wholegrain pasta and brown rice, as carbohydrates will help to fuel your training. As well as the carbohydrate, your meal should be low in fat and should not contain too much protein as this may slow down digestion and could leave you feeling uncomfortable when you run.

We recommend that you wait between one and four hours after you have eaten a meal or snack before you exercise, as this gives the body time to digest the food. Obviously the more you eat the longer the digestion process will take to set in, meaning snacks will not require a great deal of time to begin digesting, whereas a three course meal will take much longer.

Hydration

Staying well hydrated whilst exercising is crucial. When the body's water content falls below its normal level, it can have an impact on performance. If you are exercising for longer than 30 minutes then you should be drinking fluid and ideally should be keeping fluid levels topped up throughout the day. Drinking water is a good way of keeping yourself hydrated during exercise. You could also opt for energy drinks, particularly if you are undertaking endurance events such as a long run.

Many energy drinks contain electrolytes such as sodium, which help to stimulate thirst and encourage drinking, as well as enhancing the body's ability to hold water. In addition, the carbohydrates contained in many energy drinks can provide extra energy which may be needed in the latter stages of training and drinks could also provide extra protein to help prevent muscle loss.

Recovery

Eating and staying well hydrated are also essential to the training and exercise recovery process. When you have completed a training session, you should aim to have a small snack, which is rich in carbohydrates, within at least 30 minutes as this will help to promote muscle repair and growth. In addition, there are many sports drinks available which are specifically developed to aid recovery.

In order to ensure that your body is well prepared for exercise and training, understanding that different foods can provide different types of energy is important. It is also important to take into account the type and intensity of training, as this will also be a factor when determining a suitable nutrition programme.

Sports Training and Nutrition
The day-to-day diet and eating habits of people who frequently train or participate in lots of sport is very important in terms of performance level and progression. You can now tailor your diet to help you excel in your particular sport if required.

Whether you are a seasoned athlete or a beginner, and wish to optimise your performance level, a healthy and well-planned diet could help you. There is no magic food or shortcut which is going to provide your body with all of the vitamins and minerals it needs, so it is important to maintain a balanced diet incorporating a variety of food groups and nutrients. If you are interested in tailoring your nutrition to help you maximise your training potential then a qualified nutritionist could help you to do this.

Statistics on obesity, physical activity and diet: England, 2011.

Energy Bars and Gels

Energy Bars
Energy bars are usually used as a pre-run snack or for post-run recovery. You could use them on the run but few runners

find solids easy to eat on the move. However, the advantages are: they're portable and they tend to have a good balance of fast- and slow-release carbohydrate, a bit of protein for recovery and low levels of fat. See Figure 39.

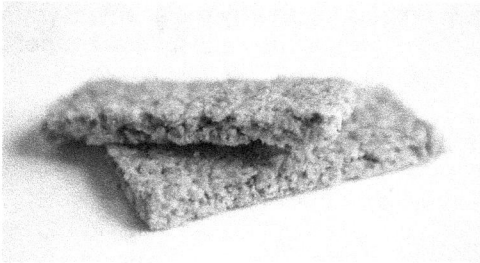

Fig. 39 Typical Energy Bar make up

How to choose an energy bar
There's a huge range of energy bars available, though the carbohydrates tend to come from similar sources: rice, oats and, in a few products, maltodextrin for complex carbohydrates, and dried fruit or fructose and glucose syrup for simple carbohydrates.

Other variants include chocolate coatings (nice, though the higher fat content makes them less digestible on the run) and high-protein bars (best for body-builders or for recovery from very high-intensity sessions). It is good practice to make sure you consume your bar with sufficient water (at least 250ml) to replace the fluids you lose in sweat, as well as to help digest the bar.

Gels
In the previous section we talked about hydration being an important part of sports nutrition. Well, Gels, like carbohydrate drinks, can provide readily and easily-absorbed

carbohydrates, often with electrolytes. Because gels contain less water than a carbohydrate drink, the carbohydrate is more concentrated and, potentially, more portable. For example, two gel sachets weighing 100g in total can contain as much carbohydrate as 1kg of carbohydrate drink. However, if you just rely on gels for energy replacement you will still need to top-up your water intake, especially in hot conditions when sweat loss will add to your fluid needs.

How to use your gel(s)

Energy gels perform the same role as carbohydrate energy drinks, because, apart from containing less water, the ingredients are almost the same. As long as you have access to extra fluid, they can be used as part of your training/racing fuelling strategy. Incidentally, most races usually have water stations, so you can consume your gel and take on some water at the same time.

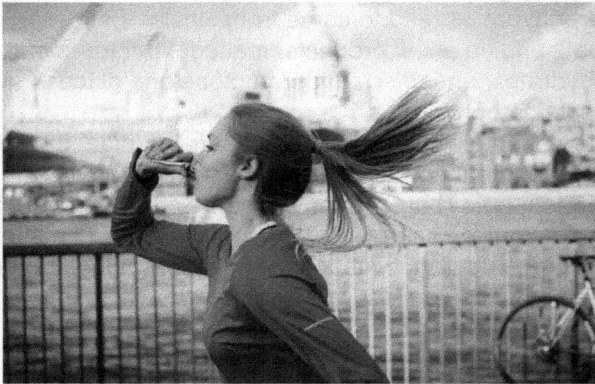

Fig. 40 Gel intake on the run. Reproduced by kind permission of Science in Sport plc

For example, if you're trying to consume 50g per hour

of carbohydrate during a race, you could either consume 800mls per hour of 6% carbohydrate drink or three gels per hour, each providing 17g of carbohydrate. You can also mix and match – for example two gels (34g of carbohydrate) plus 270mls of drink (16g of carbohydrate).

So what, actually, is inside these gel sachets?

Maltodextrin - is a carbohydrate made of glucose molecules. Maltodextrin is generally preferred to free glucose because it tends to be less sweet. It is also less likely to cause bloating and cramps, and, is effective in producing the ideal drink consistency.

Fructose - is a simple sugar derived from fruit, which provides sweetness. In combination with maltodextrin a 2:1 carbohydrate blend is produced. Compared to glucose or maltodextrin-only drinks, significantly higher rates of energy absorption can be achieved when consuming a 2:1 blend of glucose and fructose – this could be important during long runs.

Water - Although very concentrated, gels still need to contain a certain amount of water, the amount affecting both taste and consistency. Low water gels are thicker in consistency and tend to be sweeter. High water gels tend to be more liquid, leading to a more refreshing taste.

Sodium - is a key electrolyte mineral along with magnesium, calcium, potassium and chloride. Sodium is important because it not only aids the uptake of glucose from the intestine it also stimulates the desire to drink. This serves to underline the importance of consuming extra fluid along with gels especially during warmer conditions.

Citric acid - As well as providing a tangy taste, citric acid is extremely useful for ensuring that the gel product is sufficiently acidic to inhibit bacterial growth. This might be important because the liquid nature of gels means they might be more susceptible to spoilage on the shelf.

Flavouring - is vital for making the gel appetising. Natural flavourings from fruit extracts are among those most commonly used, although more exotic flavours are starting to appear on the market.

If you consume all your carbohydrate in gel form, top up with plain water rather than carbohydrate drink which would supply surplus carbohydrate. If you consume too much carbohydrate it may not be absorbed and could cause stomach upset. If you are using 2:1 glucose/fructose gels and carbohydrate drinks, you can reasonably consume up to a maximum of 80g of carbohydrate per hour, as research shows that glucose/fructose formulations are absorbed at a relatively fast rate.

Caffeine – In addition, some gels include caffeine to help prevent fatigue in longer events, like a marathon or triathlon. Like caffeinated carbohydrate drinks, gels containing caffeine are best used sparingly and towards the later stages of a longer event where the fatigue-fighting properties of caffeine are most needed. Most studies suggest that a caffeine dose of 3mg per kg of body weight is effective for fighting fatigue and prolonging endurance. **Do not exceed this amount.** Typical gel products on the market include: SiS, Powerbar, High-5 and Torq.

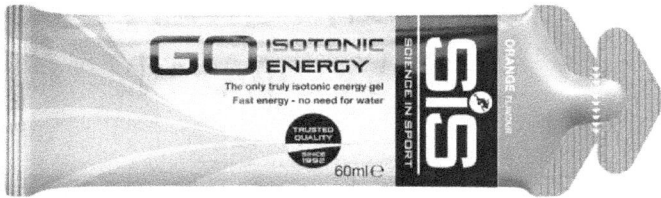

Fig. 41 Typical Gel. Reproduced by kind permission of Science in Sport plc

When Martin was competing in the UK Ironman in 2014, he had already consumed two gels whilst on the first bike lap (these gels were taped to his handlebars). Then, on lap two, thinking about topping up for the impending run, he decided to consume a 50 gramme caffeine gel. To make sure he got the full amount, he stopped his bike and tried to open the sachet. The sachet bust open and sticky gel went all over the handlebars and made a right sticky mess. Fortunately, he had one caffeine gel remaining, so he opened this, very gingerly, and consumed the full amount. There was about 20 miles to go on the bike segment and Martin said he flew round the last part of the course in order to meet the bike cut-off time.

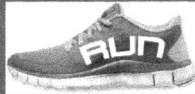

CHAPTER 9

IS IT DIFFERENT FOR WOMEN?

Introduction

Whilst the authors' are not female, they do regularly run with women athletes. However, to bring a woman's touch to the proceedings, this chapter has been developed in consultation with a leading female athlete.

In this chapter we will look at specific aspects which may apply to women. A 2012 survey (Runner's World) shows that 48% of UK runners are female (41% in the USA) so it is by no means a strictly male activity. These percentages have grown over the years, for example at the inaugural London Marathon, in 1981 only 5% of the finishers were female, whereas, in the 2015 event this had risen to 38%. Geoff and Martin surveyed their local running clubs and found that a high, and growing, proportion of members, are female.

There is sufficient medical evidence that running and fitness can bring significant benefits to women. These benefits include: reducing the effects of loss of bone density due to osteoporosis; fuelled by lowering of the hormones oestrogen and progesterone, helping to control the weight in post-menopausal women as the above hormone levels change, and easing of Pre-menstrual tension (PMT) and related conditions. Exercise has also been shown to reduce the risk of some cancers and to improve the wellbeing of cancer sufferers (in both men and women). Reference: (Journal of Clinical Oncology, 2003).

So let's start with what running gear you will need and then we will look at what issues women should be aware of, especially if you are a beginner.

Running shoes

Women's feet are different from men's, so women may need to look for running shoes which are specifically designed for them. Men's feet tend to be wider in the forefoot and heel area so running shoe manufacturers have different designs and sizes. There are however, some shoes on the market that are unisex. This is especially true of the lighter, racing type. Again, please refer to Chapter 5 for advice on how to select the best shoe type for you.

What do women wear!

Specialist running clothes can be expensive and certain manufacturers may assume that all women are a size 8 or 10 and enjoy wearing pink! However, you do not need to pay a fortune for your kit and you can still look stylish whilst pounding the pavements. You can start with a T-shirt and leggings as shown in Figure 42. The crop top and lycra shorts can come later.

Fig. 42 Women's Running Wear

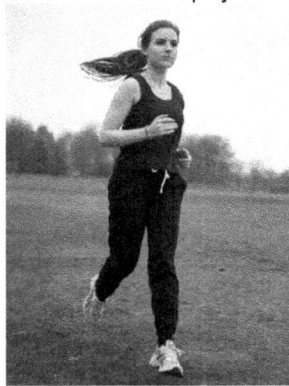

Sports bra

A woman's breasts can move around during exercise, resulting in chafing and ligament damage. Therefore, a decent sports bra is a good investment and there are plenty on the market. You will need one with good support. When buying a sports bra, it is wise to get professionally measured and take your time choosing. Figures 43a, b.

Once you are kitted out it is time to start exercising, but

first have a look at the potential issues that affect women's running, then you can be more confident when you take up exercise.

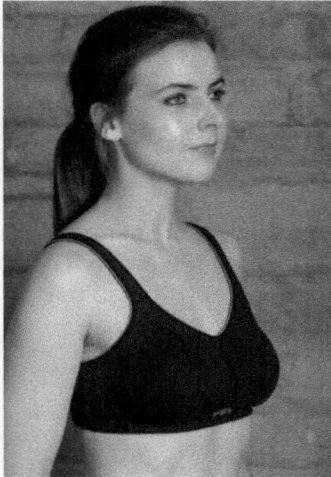 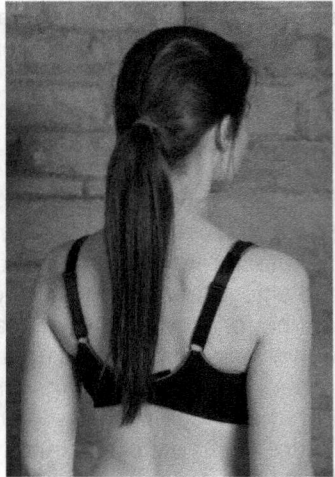

Fig. 43a   Fig. 43b

Running Safety

Feeling safe when you are out running can be more of an issue for women runners than men. Use common sense, run somewhere that is familiar to you and well-lit. Take your mobile phone, and always tell someone where you are going to run and how long you are likely to be. For additional safety, you could also take a mini alarm or, even better, run with a partner.

Time of the Month?

A woman's menstrual cycle can affect her running and not just during a period. About a week before a period starts the level of progesterone rises which increases breathing rate and can make running hard work. Body temperature also increases at this stage of the cycle. However, period cramps can actually be eased by exercise, so running during a period may not be as bad as you think. You may need to consider taking extra calcium and iron during this phase, but please consult your pharmacist.

Running during pregnancy

Running whilst pregnant needs a bit more thought and planning and a consultation with your doctor is advisable. Most women who are already regular runners should be able to continue until they find it just too uncomfortable. Figure 44.

After that, if you still want to keep up your fitness then swimming or aqua running is probably the best idea. It is not advisable to take up running from scratch during pregnancy.

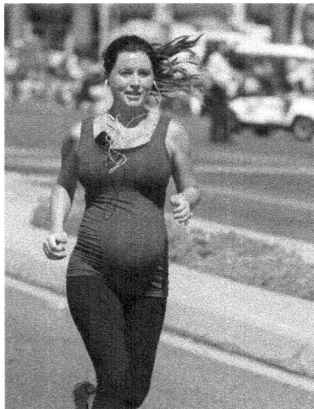

Fig. 44 Running during Pregnancy
Image with kind permission of
Nathan Rupert

As long as you have the OK from your health professional, you are aware of the warning signs of over-exertion and you carry a supply of water, you should be able to run safely during pregnancy. However, you should stop exercising immediately if you have spotting, cramping or other pains. Some doctors believe that, for women starting with a good base level of fitness, moderate exercise is not only good but could but also help to keep blood pressure in check, prevent gestational diabetes and even help women deliver closer to their due dates, often with easier deliveries.

Again, doctors would not encourage non-runners to **begin** running when they are pregnant, but they could help maintain a healthy pregnancy through walking, workouts in the pool and similar low intensity exercises. For more details on running during pregnancy, please visit: http://www.myrunningtips.com/running-while-pregnant.html

Menopause

The menopause is an important stepping stone for women and is an inevitable part of life. It occurs when the production of sex hormones decreases and monthly periods cease. In some instances menopause may be associated with adverse symptoms, although each woman's experience will be different. Natural menopause is said to have been reached when a woman has been without a period for over 12 months continuously, after which she will enter into the post-menopause. The peri-menopausal phase represents the years leading up to the final menstrual period plus the 12 months that immediately follow. In Caucasian women, the average age of menopause is between the ages of 50 and 52 years, although in some societies or ethnic groups the average age can be several years earlier.

Common symptoms of the menopause transition include

- Irregular periods, which may be heavy
- Hot flushes
- Night sweats
- Trouble sleeping

- Aches and pains
- Racing heartbeat
- Increased need to go to the toilet
- Mood changes, such as irritability or feeling low
- Trouble concentrating

Many studies, including one by the Royal College of Obstetricians and Gynaecologists*, show that exercise (alongside other measures) can help during and after menopause. Exercise can contribute to reduction/alleviation of post menopausal conditions such as: cardiovascular disease, osteoporosis, osteoarthritis and cognitive decline.
   *http://www.imsociety.org/downloads/world_menopause_day_2014/booklets/ims_wmd_booklet_2014_english.pcf

Furthermore, Sport England's **This Girl Can** campaign, which launched in January 2015, is an attempt to encourage more women into sport. This comes out of research revealing that, in the 14-40 age group, two million fewer women than men engage in sport on a regular basis and it is hoped that this and other campaigns encourage more women to take up exercise.
   In support of this, a survey by the Melpomene Institute indicated three quarters of the participants said that 'running had a positive effect' on the menopausal experience. One quarter said it eased their physical symptoms and over half felt relief from the mood and emotional symptoms.

Bone Strength
One of the biggest benefits of running for women is the effect on bone density. The depletion of oestrogen caused by the menopause normally means loss of bone density and

higher risk of osteoporosis. Running combined with strength training however, increases bone density and may reduce osteoporosis. So it is good to include strength training in your weekly schedule.

Exercise can help to alleviate Pre-menstrual (PMS) symptoms and period pain

Research by Arkansas University found that women over 30 who exercised regularly reported less cramping, bloating and breast tenderness than sedentary women, although they were not entirely symptom free.

As far as menstrual cramps are concerned, it seems that it is person-dependent as some studies show that intense training eases the pain more effectively than prolonged, gentler exercise. Whereas, a study at Dukes University, USA found that aerobic exercise was more effective at alleviating the symptoms, especially mood-related ones, than intense exercise.

Female athletes have achieved world records in all different phases of the menstrual cycle, so there's no reason why being pre-menstrual, or menstruating, should affect performance. However, when interviewed, after losing in the first round of the Australian Open tennis match in 2015, British No. 1, Heather Watson said, 'it was one of those girl things'.

Find more on menopause, PMT and period pain here: http://www.realbuzz.com/articles/exercise-and-the-menopause/#pagination-top

You can also find more specific women's running advice here: http://www.myrunningtips.com/women-running.html

CHAPTER 10

ACCESS ALL AREAS

You may have limited mobility, perhaps because of a chronic illness or condition, stiff joints, an injury or stubborn weight issues. You may be a wheelchair user or a user of other adaptability appliances. This does not mean that, to some extent, you cannot try and improve your general fitness and reap the benefits this brings (as outlined in Chapters 1 and 2).

Of course, each limited mobility condition is different and **we recommend that you talk to your health professional before embarking on a fitness programme**.

This chapter discusses ways in which you can, even with limited mobility, access fitness facilities and create a workout that suits your needs and improves your situation. In Chapter 7 you will find some basic physical movements that you can do with your upper body, lower body, or both. But first of all, you need to be able to access a suitable facility. You may be fortunate that you have access (or facilities) at home but if not here are some guidelines to support you.

How to access exercise facilities
Background

Historically, many local fitness and sports facilities were partially inaccessible for people with limited mobility. Many gyms lacked staff who were trained in disability awareness and, indeed, a number of Leisure Centres and swimming pools were 'no-go zones' for disabled people.

However, following the success of recent Paralympic Games (London 2012, Glasgow 2014 etc) and the consequent increased demand, sporting facilities are improving their access. One of the key legacy aims of the Paralympics is to increase participation in sports by Britain's 11 million disabled people. Just 18% of disabled adults undertake physical activity for more than 30 minutes a week, compared with 38% of non-disabled adults, according to Sport England.

Ideally, improvements to sports facilities will centre on key items such as:

- Wide parking bays
- Accessible changing rooms
- Suitable sports equipment
- Appropriate staff training
- Colour contrast signage
- Automatic door systems
- Swimming pool access hoist/lifts
- Seated shower areas

There are already some best-in-class facilities providing access and one example would be:
http://www.athleticbusiness.com/fitness-training/adaptive-recreation-and-fitness-facilities-set-an-example-for-all.html
This is The Virginia G. Piper Sports and Fitness Center for People with Disabilities in Phoenix, Arizona. It opened in 2012 and has a vast array of amazing facilities to accommodate ALL requirements.

In Britain, Sports facilities with suitable access for people with limited mobility are listed in the Good Access Guide:
http://www.goodaccessguide.co.uk/leisure/
This website gives details of appropriate leisure facilities by geographic region.

In addition, there is a very useful information brochure about the layout and design of leisure facilities which accommodate people with disability. This can be found at:

http://www.sportengland.org/media/30246/Accessible-Sports-Facilities-2010.pdf

User facilities
Once at the leisure facility, there is a range of equipment designed to assist people with impairment.

Typical Gym Equipment is shown in Figures 45a, b and c.

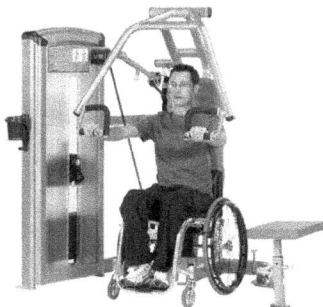

Figure 45a Total Access fitness strength press designed to be accessible to the physically impaired but which does not exclude other exercisers – Reproduced by kind permission of Cybex International UK Ltd.

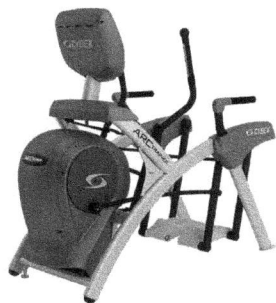

Figure 45b Total Access cardiovascular equipment designed to be accessible tc the physically impaired but which does not exclude other exercisers – Reproduced by kind permission of Cybex International UK Ltd.

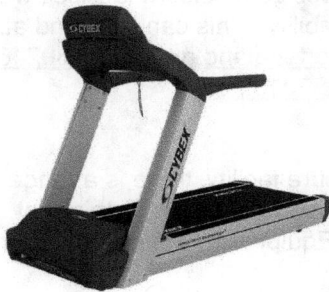

Figure 45c Total Access cardiovascular equipment designed to be accessible to the physically impaired but which does not exclude other exercisers – Designed to address the exercise needs of people with cognitive, sensory or physical disabilities, as well as the active ageing population. Multiple belt logos and colour contrasted deck and belt allow users to safely differentiate between the moving and non-moving parts. Raised console iconography and colour allows easy identification of the main controls both by colour, large buttons and text. Emergency stop lanyard provides safe emergency stop.

*Reproduced by kind permission
of Cybex International UK Ltd.*

Swimming Pool Access Hoists are also available at many modern Leisure Centres. A typical hoist is shown in Figure 46.

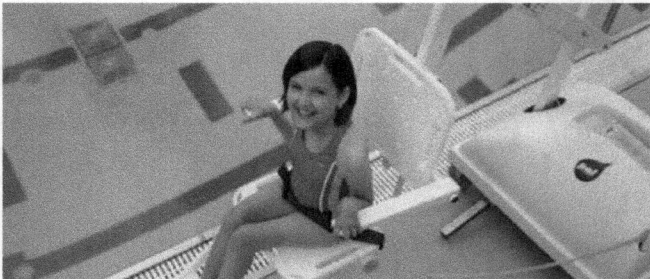

Fig. 46 Swimming Pool Access Hoist Reproduced by kind permission of Dolphin Lifts

Changing and shower areas are also well equipped to support people with varying degrees of disability, as shown in Figure 47.

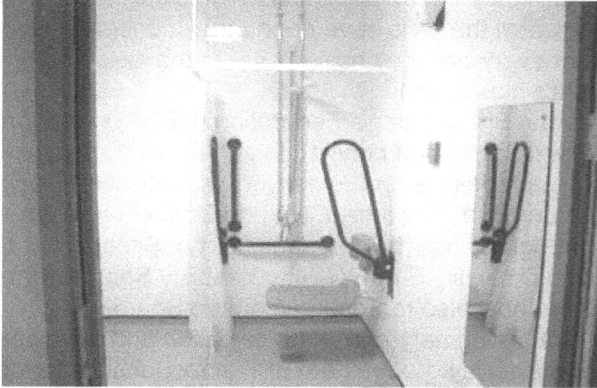

Fig. 47 Disabled Access Shower Area. Reproduced by kind permission of Henbury Leisure Centre

Alternative activities for people with disability

Boccia

Boccia is a Paralympic sport for athletes with disabilit es that have a major impact on motor skills. This target ball sport belongs to the same family as petanque and bowls. Pronounced 'Bot-cha', Boccia is a Paralympic sport introduced in 1984. Athletes throw, kick or use a ramp to propel a ball onto the court with the aim of getting closest to a 'jack' ball. It is designed specifically for athletes with a disability affecting locomotor function. It is played indoors on a court similar in size to a badminton court.

The aim of the game is to get closer to the jack than your opponent. The jack ball is white and is thrown first. One side has six red balls and the other has six blue balls. The balls are leather containing plastic granules so they don't bounce but will still roll. The side whose ball is <u>not</u> closest to the jack throws until they get a ball closest *or* until they run out of balls. Once all the balls have been thrown one side receives points for every ball they have closer to the jack than their opponent's closest ball.

The Great Britain Boccia Federation (GBBF) was formed in 2007 with the aim of bringing together the home country agencies responsible for the delivery of elite level Boccia in Great Britain at that time. CP Sport England and Wales (Boccia England now have responsibility), Scottish Disability Sport and Disability Sport Wales. Disability Sport Northern Ireland are now also represented on the Board.

The GBBF's primary role is the selection and development of the GB Boccia squad. The GBBF is responsible for sending a GB team to BISFed sanctioned international competitions to qualify teams, pairs and individuals to represent Great Britain at the Paralympic Games.

Great Britain sent a full team of nine players to the 2012 Paralympic Games in London and won two medals. David Smith won Silver in the BC1 Individual competition and the BC1/BC2 Team of Smith, Nigel Murray, Dan Bentley and Zoe Robinson won Bronze.

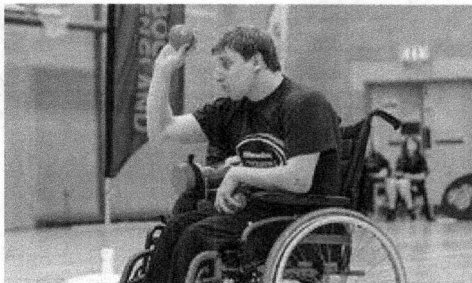

Fig. 48 Athlete playing Boccia - Reproduced by kind permission of Boccia England.

New Age Kurling

New Age Kurling is a form of the original curling game, but adapted so that it can be played indoors on any smooth, flat surface, such as a sports hall, rather than on ice. Importantly, the game can be played by both able-bodied and disabled people of all ages alike. It has become so popular that it is recognised by most disabled unions in the United Kingdom and is fast becoming a mainstream sport in schools and after school clubs. This can be a competitive sport but will also be well accepted, and thoroughly enjoyed, by all that play. This new sport is now played in 47 countries around the world. New Age Kurling falls into all the government guidelines for exercise and bringing sport into schools.

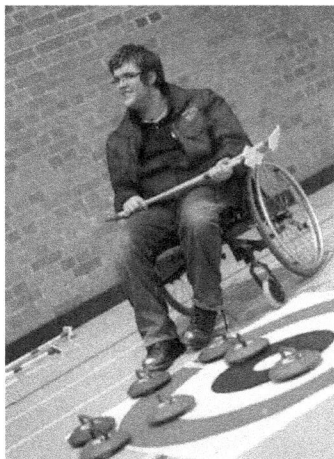

Fig. 49 Kurling competitor - reproduced by kind permission of New Age Kurling.

Cycling Opportunities

Medical proof shows that an active person will maintain a greater independence and a healthier life style and this is crucial for mobility impaired people. Non-impact exercise such as cycling, coupled with the correct assistance, training and equipment, will improve a person's health and well-being.

"Aerodynamically, the bumble bee shouldn't be able to fly, but the bumble bee doesn't know it so goes on flying anyway."
– Mary Kay Ash

One such organisation to have spearheaded this form of exercise is 'Empowered people'. This is a registered charity whose aim is to enable all adults with disabilities, from all backgrounds regardless of gender, race or level of ability, to improve their health and wellbeing through cycling. Together with other activities providing the correct tools, support and encouragement, enabling people to achieve their personal targets. This charity also aims to help change public preconceptions about disability and promote the potential of all persons of restricted abilities.

The charity organises and runs cycling events. Selected riders of varying disability take part in these organised events throughout the year. A personalised training programme brings disabled riders' endurance up to a level that allows them to ride in various prestigious events throughout the UK. The EMpowered team consists of a group of individuals who have been brought together by their love and passion for cycling. They are ordinary people who have had to adapt their lives on a daily basis and are ready to prove what can be achieved. These are inclusive and fully supported rides for people who are over eighteen years of age.

http://www.empoweredpeople.co.uk/

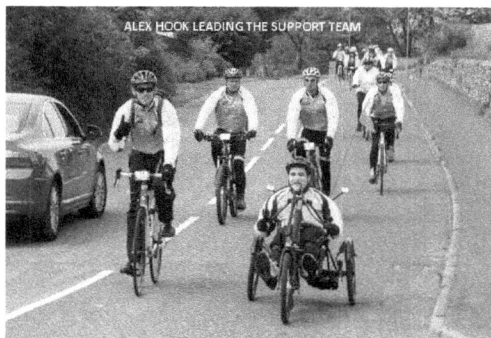

Fig. 50 Empowered people in action
Reproduced by kind permission of EMpowered people.

CHAPTER 11

A Wonderful Uplifting Experience – Racing

Turning your training into competition

Can you imagine crossing the finishing line of a race that you set as your goal a few months before? Well, it can actually come true. For Geoff and Martin there is nothing better than pinning-on a race number at the start of an event. It can be a little scary but always well worthwhile.

Races generally cater for all levels of ability. Racing helps to improve your fitness and style and is a great way to build relationships with a wider circle of runners.

There are many different kinds of running events from fun runs, 5k park runs (which, incidentally, are free to enter. Please refer to www.parkrun.org.uk) right up to ultra-distance challenges. Races take place on road, trail, fell or track and some combine a number of these within the event. Popular race events can be found on web sites, such as www.Ukresults.co.uk , many of which are listed in the Reference section at the end of this book and in running magazines such as: *Athletics Weekly*, *Runner's World* and most running club websites.

For races in USA, go to www.runningintheusa.com.

To find races in Europe, you could try www.runningfgrance or www.mynextrun.com.

Figures 51 and 52 show, respectively, Geoff at the Berlin Marathon and his wife, Sarah, at the Guernsey Marathon.

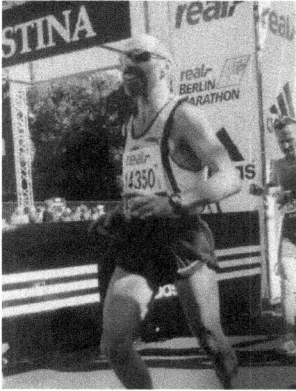
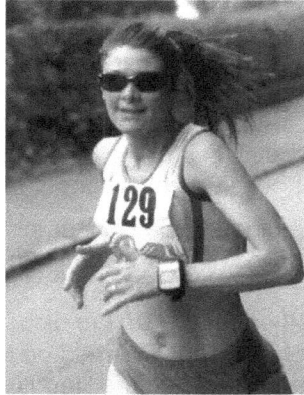

Fig. 51 Geoff at the Berlin Marathon   Fig. 52 Sarah at the Guernsey Marathon.

You may find that as you increase the number of events you do, you will have favourites that you return to year after year, sometimes to set a new course record or achieve a personal goal. You may also return because it has beer a good sociable club event, or often for reasons not to do with running i.e. childhood memories, a good holiday etc.

Entering a race is a relatively easy process, made easier by many races now offering an on line entry system. Alternatively, fill out a paper entry which can usually be picked up at races or downloaded from the club web site. Many races allow entry on the day (there may a higher fee on the day), but always check to see if the race has not become full.

Age is no barrier

Being middle aged does not prevent you from improving and can allow latent ability to be recognised on a wider stage.

There are web sites such as 'The *Power of 10*' http://www.thepowerof10.info/ that can show how you are doing against others in your age group. Geoff, for example was 1st in his age group in the London Marathon. The ageing process does not exclude you from being competitive and competition can be very satisfying. Being older does not prevent you from beating those considerably younger than yourself.

The oldest male finisher in the London Marathon was Fauja Singh who, in 2004, completed the 26.2 mile course in 6 hours 7 minutes at the age of 93. His run at the 2011 Toronto Marathon made him the oldest ever marathon finisher at the age of 100. Singh carried on running until he was 101 after he had completed the Hong Kong 10km in 1:32:28. At the age of 92, Gladys Burrill became the oldest female marathon finisher. She completed the Honolulu Marathon in 2010, in a time of 9:53. Interestingly, she did not run her first marathon until she was 86.

In 2013, **79 year old** Harriet Anderson became the oldest woman to ever finish the IRONMAN Triathlon World Championship. This race consisted of a 2.4-mile swim, followed by a 112-mile bike ride, topped off with a 26.2-mile marathon run. Anderson fell off her bike during the latter stages of the ride but despite a few bruises, she got back on her bike and finished the course before the cut off time of 17 hours. She got to the finish line in 16 hours and 56 minutes to take the age group record. Figure 53.

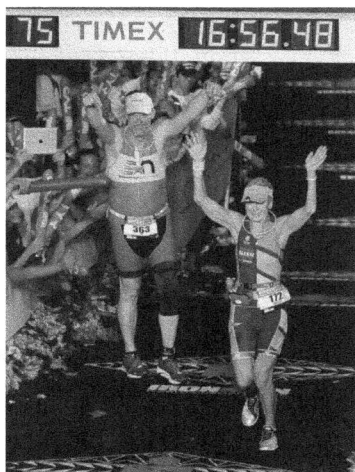

Fig. 53 Harriet Anderson, aged 78, finishing the Ironman Triathlon. Reproduced by kind permission of Harriet Anderson.

Becoming more experienced – the World is your Oyster
When you become more experienced at running and have more confidence with your style, pace etc, you can start to experiment with various types of events.

From a running perspective you can train on, and enter races on, the track, road, trail and fell. Around the country and around the world, there are many races you can compete in at all levels and at many distances.

Alternative, related events
After a while many runners like to try their hand at cycling and swimming. These two sports, whilst they don't suit everybody, can actually complement your running.

Swimming - allows you to exercise (especially cardiovascular) without having your body weight bearing down on your lower limb joints. Swimming can be a useful means to obtaining fitness and can form part of a cross training regime. If you are new to swimming, or not a good swimmer, don't be turned off. Lessons are normally available at most public swimming pools and you can complete your own sessions, similar to those you might do at a running club. As with running, the kit required for swimming has minimal cost.

Cycling - Cycling also gives you a fresh perspective on exercise, can help you to recover from injury and allows you to cover many miles and enjoy lovely scenery in a relatively short time. Cycling can be very sociable and many cyclists stop along the route for a cake and coffee. Please ensure that your bicycle is roadworthy and that you wear the appropriate safety equipment, **especially a helmet**.

Please visit British Cycling Go Sky ride www.goskyride.com to find local, guided rides, in your area.

Triathlon - Both swimming and cycling can then, of course, be used IN CONJUNCTION with running by entering a triathlon. This event combines all the above disciplines and helps with spreading the physical load, can be a good exercise diversion and may bring new interest to your sport. It may require some planning and rethinking of your training, but can be very rewarding.

There is also, in effect, a fourth part to the triathlon event which is the transition. This takes place when going from one discipline to the next i.e. swim-to-bike, which may be strange at first but with a bit of personal organisation is very achievable.

The triathlon, like running, comes in different distances. The most common distances are known as sprint events, which usually incorporate a 400metre pool swim, a 20km cycle ride and a 5km run.

These are usually easy to do and take place from a local leisure centre. Olympic distance triathlons have a 1500metre open water swim, a 40km cycle ride and a10km run with transitions between each discipline. Also, there are longer distance triathlons, like the Ironman, for the more adventurous, see Figure 54.

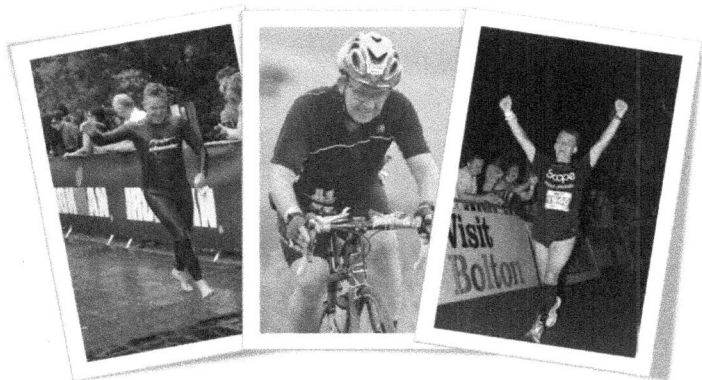

Fig. 54 Martin at the 2014 UK IRONMAN event

Entering triathlons is the same process as a running event but will probably cost more in order to cover the more complex organisation required.

Taking sport and fitness even further
If you wish to be more adventurous, or you just fancy having a go at different sports, you can go to the BBC Get Inspired Website. http://www.bbc.co.uk/sport/get-inspired

On this website, you can enter your postcode and the site will reveal all the different sporting opportunities in your area. This could be trampolining, archery, netball and many other exciting activities as shown in Figure 55.

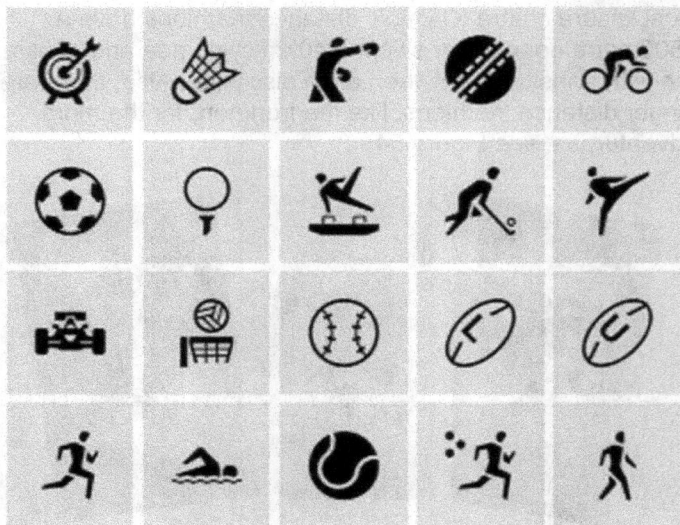

Fig. 55 Sporting Opportunities available via the BBC 'Get Inspired Website'.

However eager and enthusiastic you might be, please do not be tempted to ride a bicycle without wearing a suitable helmet.

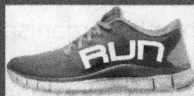

CHAPTER 17

Giving is Better than Receiving – Running for a Charity

You may have seen on TV, the many thousands of runners in large scale running events like the London Marathon and Great North Run, where the majority of the field is represented by people raising money to support the many worthy causes. Running for charity is not everybody's cup of tea but, if this appeals to you then there are many opportunities to run in popular races by taking a charity (or Gold Bond) place. http://www.runforcharity.com/find-a-charity/golden-bond-places.html

Usually, you will be required to raise a minimum amount for your chosen charity but you do get very good support from your charity and it is a great way to meet new, like-minded, people. If you choose to run for charity you may need to be aware of your obligations to them. You will need to raise awareness for your cause, carry-out the fundraising and collect the donations. This all takes time and energy which may detract from your training schedule.

There are many ways to raise funds; rattling a bucket in the high street or knocking on neighbours' doors. But the most common way of fundraising is through the internet. Typically, if you are accepted for a Gold Bond place, the host charity will normally set up your Just Giving page for you. This enables you to e-mail, or Facebook, a bunch of friends and they can sponsor you for your cause by following an embedded link in your e-mail.

On your Just Giving page you can build your profile, include a photo, discuss why your charity is important to you and include your automatic 'thank you' message. A graphic shows how close to / or how much you have exceeded your target by.

Of course you don't have to feel compelled to raise thousands of pounds by entering mass participation events like the London Marathon. You can raise more modest amounts, e.g. for your local church or youth club, and again use the internet as a communications vehicle.

You can set up your own Just Giving or Local Giving page by going to JustGiving.com and following the instructions. Your page could look something like Figure 56.

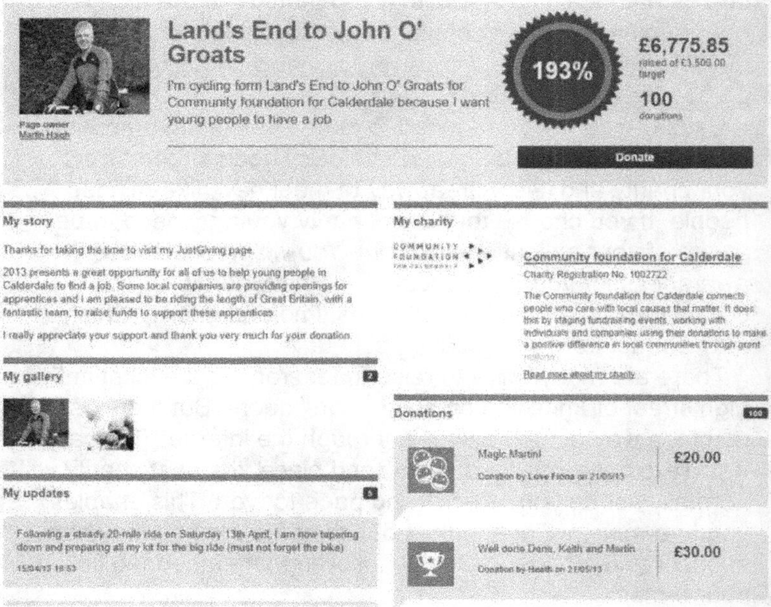

Land's End to John O' Groats

I'm cycling form Land's End to John O' Groats for Community foundation for Calderdale because I want young people to have a job

Page owner
Martin Haigh

193%

£6,775.85
raised of £3,500.00 target

100
donations

Donate

My story

Thanks for taking the time to visit my JustGiving page.

2013 presents a great opportunity for all of us to help young people in Calderdale to find a job. Some local companies are providing openings for apprentices and I am pleased to be riding the length of Great Britain, with a fantastic team, to raise funds to support these apprentices.

I really appreciate your support and thank you very much for your donation.

My gallery

My updates

Following a steady 20-mile ride on Saturday 13th April, I am now tapering down and preparing all my kit for the big ride (must not forget the bike).

15/04/13 18:53

My charity

COMMUNITY FOUNDATION

Community foundation for Calderdale
Charity Registration No. 1002722

The Community foundation for Calderdale connects people who care with local causes that matter. It does this by staging fundraising events, working with individuals and companies using their donations to make a positive difference in local communities through grant making.

Read more about my charity

Donations

	Magic Martini Donation by Love Fiona on 21/05/13	£20.00
	Well done Denis, Keith and Martin Donation by Health on 21/05/13	£30.00

Fig. 56 Just Giving Page Layout example

In 2013, Martin cycled from Land's End to John O' Groats and raised funds through Just Giving. He was with a team of seven riders who set up a Group Page to show the cumulative amount raised for the charity. Also, in 2014, Martin raised funds for SCOPE charity by using a Virgin Money Giving Page.

It is important to note that Just Giving and Local Giving takes a small percentage to cover their administration costs, but using their facilities can save you a lot of time and energy by centralising your collection point. You can use this time and energy for your training so your fundraising run, swim or bike ride is an enjoyable experience and not a chore.

Regulations around charitable donations and the UK Tax position – Often a UK Tax payer can claim Gift Aid which means that an extra 25% of your donation is given to your charity. Your donors must ensure that their postcode is entered on the donation page or form.

Here is a sample of the popular National charities that are geared-up to offer places.

Cancer Research UK – one day we will beat cancer – www.cancerreasearchuk.org

British Heart Foundation – research into heart disease www.bhf.org.uk

Mencap – a leading learning disability charity – www.mencap.org.uk

SCOPE – helping families with disability www.scope.og.uk

Guidedogs for the Blind – a charity that supports people who are fully or partially sighted – www.guidedogs.org.uk

Bowel Cancer - https://www.beatingbowelcancer.org

Macmillan Cancer Support – www.Macmillan.org.uk

You may also have your own local cause, such as: **Overgate Hospice** www.overgatehospice.org.uk

The brands of the charities mentioned are shown in Figure 57.

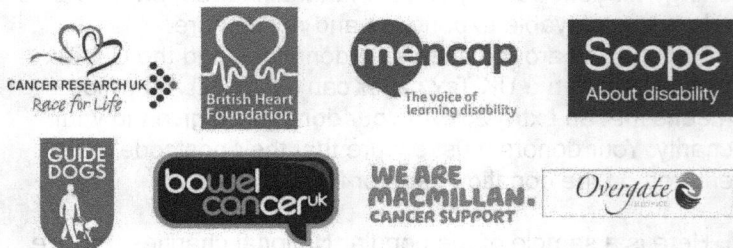

Fig. 57 Charity Brands

Spare Copy of your Fitness Goal Wheel is shown in Figure 58.
On a scale of 0 to 10, where are you today? Why not complete the wheel below to see where you might want to place your emphasis.

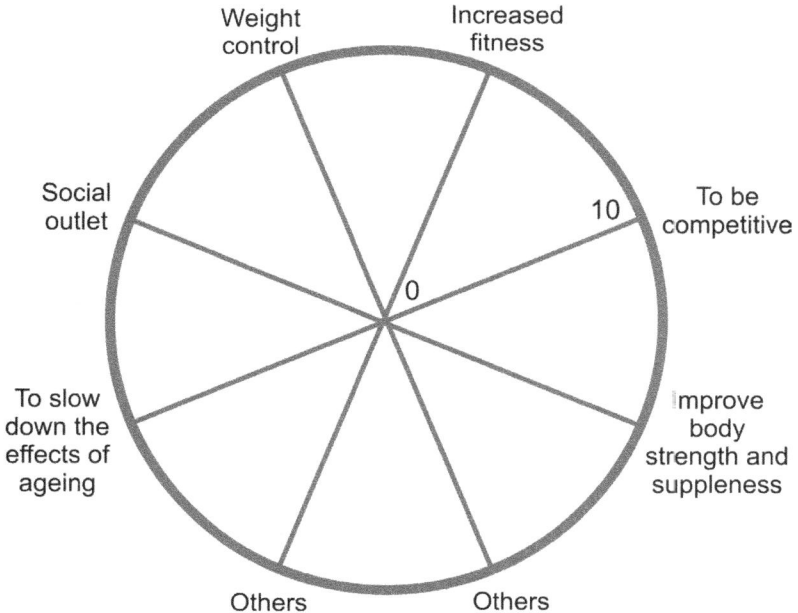

Fig. 58 Running Goals Wheel (2nd copy)

As you can see, each segment is labelled to represent possible beneficial effects from running. With **0** in the centre and **10** on the outside edge of the circle, rate your current level of satisfaction for each area by making a mark along each of the lines. There are a couple of 'others' or blank areas where you can add your own categories. You may even wish to select one from the cloud inside the front cover of this book.

Then look at the circle and ask 'if I have to select one area on which to focus, which would it be in terms of giving me the highest impact or biggest benefit from running? You don't have to pick the category with the lowest score. For the selected category alone, clearly identify what '10' will be like (when you are satisfied with improvements here). This is your **Inspirational Running Goal.**

If you are re-visiting this wheel, you can now add-in your achieved goals, perhaps using a different coloured pen.

References
Running Clubs in UK
To find a running club near you, you can go to the British Athletics website and enter your postcode. Please follow the link: http://www.britishathletics.org.uk/grassroots/search/

Sports shops in UK
There are many sports shops in UK and these include:
Sportsshoes www.sportsshoes.com
Sweatshop www.sweatshop.co.uk
Runnersneed www.runnersneed.com
Women's sports shop www.very.co.uk
Up and Running www.upandrunning.co.uk
Wiggle www.wiggle.co.uk

Popular UK races
There are many opportunities for you to find a race in your locality and you might wish to visit the UK Results site www.ukresults.net

Popular USA Races

New York Marathon http://www.tcsnycmarathon.org/
Chicago Marathon http://www.chicagomarathon.com/
Boston Marathon http://www.baa.org/races/boston-marathon.
aspx

Popular races in Europe

Paris to Versailles run http://marathons.ahotu.com/event/
paris-versailles
Berlin Marathon http://www.bmw-berlin-marathon.com/en/
Rome Marathon http://www.maratonadiroma.it/?lang=en

AIMS

The official site for International Marathon and Distance
Races. Any race listed on this site guarantees that the
distance is accurately measured. http://aimsworldrunning.org/
Calendar.htm

Using Technology to Enhance your Running and Fitness Experience

Electronic technology is part of everyday life and, when used appropriately, can complement your fitness experience. Typical technologies include: **Wearable's** (with Heart Rate Monitor, GPS and workout logging), **Mobile phones** (with Apps for iPhone or Android), **Tablets** or **PC-based** exercise planning and monitoring software.

With the help of Apps for your iPhone, Andriod device or Tablet, you can enhance your running and fitness experience and use these tools to help keep track of your progress. In this Appendix, a selection of devices and the current popular Apps have been highlighted. There is a plethora of technology available and, we recognise that new items are coming onto the market all the time. So, for the latest Apps and gadgets, you could visit your local high street retailer or browse the internet.

Whilst these smart aids are helpful, it is not advisable to rely on them as your only way of planning a route, recording your time or finding out how your body has performed. For your running to be beneficial, it is important to be aware of your surroundings and to understand how your body is reacting to exercise, from your own feelings, and not what your device might say. Remember that on your run, your device may lose connectivity and could then provide you with misleading or inaccurate information. Also, please ensure that the App is compatible with your device.

Wearables

The type of running watch or GPS sports watch used is very much down to personal choice and depends on the amount of detail you want from your fitness activity. This depends on whether you are interested in something to track your jogging, or to provide advanced information that will help you achieve your PB. Beyond just simple tracking and pace information, the latest watches on the market can provide heart rate information, or even, detailed observations of your running style.

Some wearable's are expensive, some are more affordable. Most have GPS capability and a few have full mapping. There are a few with heart rate monitors built in and selected ones that cater for swimming and cycling needs as well.

A selection is given in this appendix.

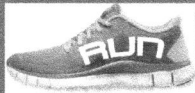

If you feel the need to wear headphones, please be aware that this will impair your spatial awareness (you may not be able to hear runners, cyclists or traffic around you). In addition, some race organisers strictly forbid the wearing of headphones during an event.

As with the use of headphones, we recommend that you take extra care when you have a mobile device with you.

Do not be tempted to glance at your screen when you are about to cross a busy road.

Apple Watch - This device released in 2015, confirms that fitness isn't just about running, biking or hitting the gym. It's also about being active throughout the day. Apple Watch measures all the ways you move, such as walking the dog, taking the stairs or playing with your children. It even keeps track of when you stand up, and encourages you to keep moving. Because it all counts and it all adds up.

http://www.apple.com/uk/watch/

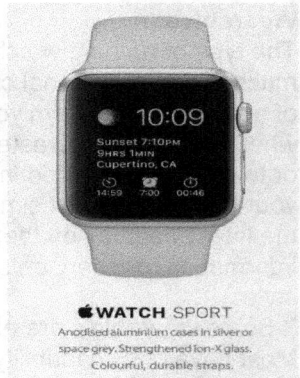

WATCH SPORT
Anodised aluminium cases in silver or space grey. Strengthened Ion-X glass. Colourful, durable straps.

The TomTom Sport App - lets you connect a TomTom GPS running watch directly to a MapMyRun account. It is then possible to synchronise your runs, including distance, pace and heart rate information to keep track of relevant statistics.

http://www.tomtom.com/en_gb/sports/multi-sport/

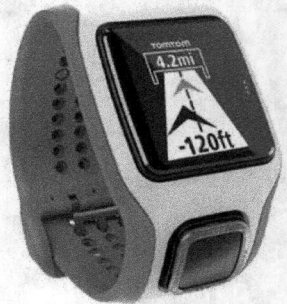

Garmin - has an extensive range of wearable devices and, some are designed to be an all-in-one fitness solution rather than purely a running watch.

The Garmin Forerunner 15, for example, tracks you while you're hitting the streets and seated at your desk.

The built-in GPS gives you distance and pace and you can hook up a range of other external sensors including heart rate monitors, cycle sensors and foot pads that measure additional statistics like how many steps you've taken, calories and treadmill runs. It's also waterproof to 50m enabling swimming sessions. It has 8 hours battery life in GPS mode or five weeks in activity tracking mode, and all of the data can be synchronised and scrutinised via the Garmin Connect smartphone app and web tools.

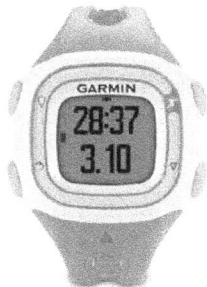

www.garmin.com

Apps for iPhone, Android and tablets

S Health - This is an application on Samsung Android devices and it allows you to manage your health, set fitness goals, check your progress and keep track of your overall health.

https://shealth.samsung.com/

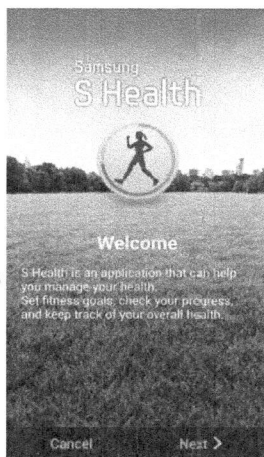

RunKeeper - can be used on Android and iPhone and uses the built-in GPS technology to track your fitness adventures. It has a very easy to use interface and you can use it to monitor running, walking, cycling and many other activities too. You can also enter activities manually; if you do your exercise on your treadmill, RunKeeper still has you covered. RunKeeper syncs up to its own web portal where you can view your history and stats in more detail. Integration with Facebook and Twitter is also included.

www.Runkeeper.com

Strava GPS Cycling and Running App - lets you track your running and riding with GPS, join Challenges, share photos from your activities, and follow friends.

www.strava.com

PC-Based fitness/route planning software

MapMyRide and MapMyRun - can be used to track routes, speed, distance, elevation, calories, time and more and there are audio alerts to update you on your progress. The sister application, **MapMyRun** works in a very similar way and is great for planning running routes and checking routes following a run.

   www.mapmyrun.com

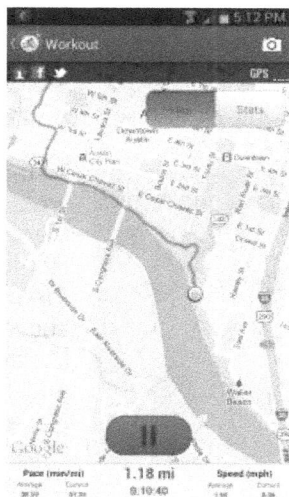

*G*eoff and Martin like to use MapMyRun for planning or checking routes after a run and they use Strava on their road bikes.

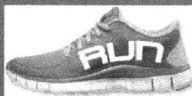

About the Authors

Dr. Martin Haigh

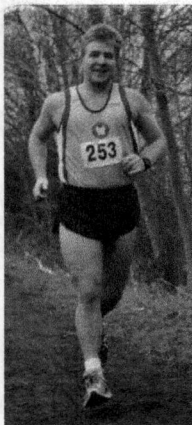

– started running at the age of 20 after a footballing injury put him out of that sport. Martin has been a member of Halifax Harriers for 42 years. He is their Vice President and former Chairman of their successful Race Committee. He has run 20 Marathons (four of them under three hours) and 10 consecutive Yorkshire Three Peaks Races (five of them under 3:30). Each Marathon has been completed to raise funds for charities, such as: Whizz Kids, Outward Bound Trust, Cancer Research, St. John's Ambulance, Calderdale Special Care Baby Unit, Bermerside Special School in Halifax and Children with Leukaemia. Martin has also competed in many other races; on the fells, trail and on the track. Martin is a Triathlete and has competed in many events including the London Triathlon and, in July 2014, completed the IRONMAN UK, raising funds for SCOPE in the process. Also in 2013 Martin cycled 950 miles, from Land's End to John O' Groats, to raise money for the apprentice charity Cycle for Work, (now Working Wonders). Martin is a British Cycling, Sky Ride Leader and a UK Athletics Leader in Running Fitness.

Geoff Cumber

– started running at the age of 38 and very quickly joined a running club. Since then he has trained in a very focused way which has enabled him to run 37 Marathons with 18 of them under three hours and also has a best 10k time of 38 minutes (at the age of 61). Geoff has competed on a global stage and has won many prizes in the over 55, over 60 and over 65 category. He won his age group, at the London Marathon in 2007, with a time of 2 hours 53 minutes (which was a course record for seven years) followed, in 2008, by winning his age group in the Boston (USA) Marathon, the world's oldest event at this distance. Geoff has been the 6th fastest Marathon runner, for his age, in the world. He is the third fastest in Europe and quickest in the UK. Geoff has also competed in 15 Triathlons and has picked up prizes in various categories. Geoff has been a member of Halifax Harriers since 1992 and puts a lot back into the sport. He is a founder member of the Harriers Race Committee and has been Race Director for a number of high-profile events. Geoff is married to Sarah Cumber who is also a seriously fast runner and 17th Lady in the London Marathon in 2014.

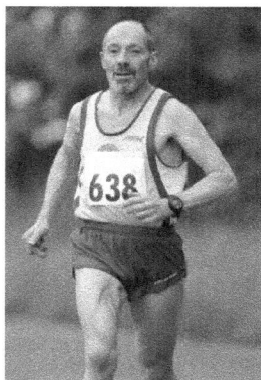

Index

O

obesity 3, 9, 109, 116
One Leg Squat 83, 84
osteoarthritis 14, 127

P

pain management 5
parkrun 138
Patellar tendinitis 104
Pectoralis 78
Piriformis 79
Plantar fasciitis 103
posture 9, 14, 16, 32, 50, 62, 75, 88, 105
Power of 10 140
pregnancy 125, 126
Pre-menstrual tension 122
Press-Ups 85
Pronation 45
protein 18, 29, 113, 115, 117

Q

quadriceps 50, 78, 82, 83, 104

R

Racing 47, 127, 138
Racing flat 47

S

T

U

V

W

www.ingramcontent.com/pod-product-compliance
Lightning Source LLC
Chambersburg PA
CBHW072144270326
41931CB00010B/1886